# MONOCULAR SURGERY

## Esotropia

| MR Recession | LR Resection |
|---|---|
| $15^\Delta$ - 3.0 mm | 3.5 mm |
| $20^\Delta$ - 3.5 mm | 4.0 mm |
| $25^\Delta$ - 4.0 mm | 5.0 mm |
| $30^\Delta$ - 4.5 mm | 5.5 mm |
| $35^\Delta$ - 5.0 mm | 6.0 mm |
| $40^\Delta$ - 5.5 mm | 6.5 mm |
| $50^\Delta$ - 6.0 mm | 7.0 mm |
| $60^\Delta$ - 6.5 mm | 7.5 mm |
| $70^\Delta$ - 7.0 mm | 8.0 mm |

## Exotropia

| LR Recession | MR Resection |
|---|---|
| $15^\Delta$ - 4.0 mm | 3.0 mm |
| $20^\Delta$ - 5.0 mm | 4.0 mm |
| $25^\Delta$ - 6.0 mm | 4.5 mm |
| $30^\Delta$ - 6.5 mm | 5.0 mm |
| $35^\Delta$ - 7.0 mm | 5.5 mm |
| $40^\Delta$ - 7.5 mm | 6.0 mm |
| $50^\Delta$ - 8.5 mm | 6.5 mm |

# Color Atlas of Strabismus Surgery

Third Edition

# Color Atlas of Strabismus Surgery

## Strategies and Techniques

Kenneth W. Wright, MD
*Director, Wright Foundation for Pediatric Ophthalmology and Strabismus*
*Director of Pediatric Ophthalmology, Cedars-Sinai Medical Center,*
  *Los Angeles*
*Visiting Associate in Chemical Engineering, California Institute of*
  *Technology*
*Clinical Professor of Ophthalmology, USC Keck School of Medicine*
*Los Angeles, California, USA*

Editor
Sonal Farzavandi, FRCS (Edin)
*Senior Consultant*
*Pediatric Ophthalmology and Strabismus Service*
*Singapore National Eye Centre*
*National University Hospital*
*Singapore*

Reviewer
Lisa Thompson, MD
*Consulting Physician*
*Stroger Hospital of Cook County*
*Chicago, Illinois, USA*

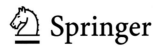 Springer

Kenneth W. Wright, MD
Director, Wright Foundation for Pediatric Ophthalmology and Strabismus
Director of Pediatric Ophthalmology, Cedars-Sinai Medical Center, Los Angeles
Visiting Associate in Chemical Engineering, California Institute of Technology
Clinical Professor of Ophthalmology, USC Keck School of Medicine
Los Angeles, CA, USA
www.wrighteyecare.com

Library of Congress Control Number: 2006925855

ISBN-10: 0-387-33249-9
ISBN-13: 978-0-387-33249-9

Printed on acid-free paper.

9 8 7 6 5 4 3 2 1

springer.com

# Preface to the Third Edition

Strabismus can be devastating to our patients, yet often difficult to treat even for the seasoned veteran. The goal of the *Atlas of Strabismus Surgery* is to clearly and succinctly share with the reader strategies and surgical techniques that will improve the care of our patients. The atlas covers the management of wide range of strabismus disorders from the relatively simple horizontal strabismus to complex cyclovertical deviations. A variety of surgical techniques are presented, starting with the simple basics and progressing to complicated surgical techniques, such as the delicate superior oblique tendon expander procedure, nd the retrieval of a slipped/lost rectus muscle. The atlas is designed to help surgeons of diverse experience, from the resident ophthalmologist to the most experienced strabismologist.

The third edition underwent a true makeover, with virtually every chapter receiving significant changes. Examples include a section on "Planning for Success" to Chapter 2 that provides a logical approach to forming a treatment plan. Incomitant strabismus and torticollis associated with nystagmus or strabismus can be challenging to treat, so we have added a chapter specifically dealing with these important disorders. Throughout the book, clinical case examples have been added to illustrate strabismus treatment strategies. Relatively new to most strabismus surgeons is the use of topical anesthesia for strabismus surgery. Topical anesthesia strabismus surgery requires special techniques to avoid patient discomfort, and a chapter has been added on this up-and-coming procedure. The book has been updated to reflect changes in choice of suture materials, such as the use of nonabsorbable suture for inferior rectus recession. We are also introducing several new titanium instruments from Titan Surgical Company that improve the efficiency and safety of strabismus surgery.

As in previous editions, color photographs are paired with line drawings to help explain the surgical techniques. The simplicity of the line drawing helps to teach technique, while the photographs add the reality of surgical field. This format innovated by the author in the first edition won a publishers award in Philadelphia. To even further improve on this winning format, the third edition has a companion DVD with more than ten videos of strabismus surgery. This combination of line drawings, color photographs, and surgical videos provides the student with the next best thing to live surgery.

I would like to give a special thanks to my dear friend Sonal Farzavandi, MD, for her tenacity in editing every line of text, checking each index entry, and helping with the content. Without Sonal's help this project would still be lingering today. Lisa Thompson, MD, one of my outstanding fellows also deserves a sincere thanks for her encouragement and for helping with editing of the book. It is my sincere hope that the third edition will help the surgeon better manage strabismus, improve patient outcomes, and make the great field of strabismus even more rewarding.

Kenneth W. Wright, MD

# Preface to the Second Edition

The second edition of the *Color Atlas of Ophthalmic Surgery—Strabismus* is an updated version of the original award-winning textbook published in 1991. The new atlas retains the same style of simplicity and clarity of the first edition. In addition, we have added a new section, "Management Strategies", which includes seven chapters on the practical management of strabismus sydromes. The idea is to provide the reader with a concise synopsis of what to do for a specific type of strabismus. Section two details strabismus surgical techniques and has been extensively revised and updated from the original edition. Chapter 22, "Reoperation Techniques" was added and describes the management of slipped/lost muscles and strabismus after retinal detachment surgery. As in the first edition, the section on surgical techniques combines line drawings and color photographs of actual surgery to offer both simplicity and realism required for teaching new techniques. I hope you will find this new edition useful in your strabismus practice.

I would like to add a special thanks to Tina Kiss, our pediatric ophthalmology administrator, for her many long hours and weekends without which this project would not have come to fruition. I would also like to extend my sincere gratitude to Laura Bonsall for her encouragement to pursue this project and for her expertise and creativity in the layout and formatting of this book. In addition, I would like to acknowledge all of my fellows who have influenced the material in this book, especially Peter Spiegel, Dean Bonsall, and Gabriela Salvador for their thorough review of the manuscript. Finally, I would like to recognize Allergan, Bausch & Lomb Surgical, Ethicon, Discovery Fund for Eye Research, Cedars-Sinai Medical Center, and University of California, Irvine for their unselfish support.

Kenneth Weston Wright, MD

# Preface to the First Edition

The Strabismus volume of Color Atlas of Ophthalmic Surgery was written as a practical text to teach strabismus surgical technique. The best surgical training is obviously hands-on experience; however, a surgical reference is critical to prepare the novice student for the surgical experience, and also for the veteran surgeon to review or expand his surgical repertoire. No drawing can capture the true appearance of the surgical scene, yet a photograph lacks the simplicity which is necessary for the teaching of a surgical procedure. Our strategy was to provide both line drawings and photographs of actual surgery to provide the most realistic presentation yet with the simplicity necessary for teaching new techniques.

Teaching surgical technique is the major goal of this atlas; however, background information, such as muscle physiology and indications for surgery, is provided when applicable. The atlas is intended to be a "how-to" book, and to describe in detail the most effective specific surgical procedures rather than present a short overview of every surgical procedure. Throughout the atlas, surgical drawings and photographs present the surgeon's view, with the upper lid at the bottom and lower lid at the top. The drawings and photographs of surgical procedures show the left eye unless otherwise stated.

The author would like thank the other contributors, Dr. Laurie Christensen, Dr. Michael Repka, Dr. Burton Kushner, Dr. Monte Del Monte and Dr. Malcolm Mazow for their excellent work. Acknowledgement must also go to Dr. Marshall M. Parks and Dr. David L. Guyton, under whom I was fortunate enough to train. Much of the material in this volume has come either directly or indirectly from their brilliant and innovative work. I would also like to express my sincere gratitude to the fellows who have so greatly influenced and improved my own surgical techniques: Doctors Andrea Lanier, Laurie Christensen, John McVey, and Andrew Terry. I would like to extend special thanks to Dr. Byng-Moo Min and Dr. Chan Park, visiting research fellows from Korea, and to Dr. Ann U. Stout, for their expert review of the manuscript. Finally, I would like to acknowledge the contributions from Margaret Brown-Multani, Surgical Technician, Children's Hospital of Los Angeles; Paula Edelman, C.O., Children's Hospital of Los Angeles, for clinical support; and from my sister, Lisa Wright, for her long hours of editing, revising, and re-revising the manuscript.

Too often, strabismus surgery is referred to as "easy", and is often delegated in training programs to first-year residents. Strabismus surgery is easy when performed properly; however, the untrained surgeon has the potential to do more harm than good. It is the author's sincere hope that this atlas will improve strabismus surgical techniques and ultimately benefit patients with strabismus.

Kenneth Weston Wright, MD

# Acknowledgment

Thanks to the supporters of Wright Foundation for Pediatric Ophthalmology and Strabismus who help us with our mission:

*To reduce blindness and suffering from eye disorders in infants and children and to improve the treatment of strabismus through research, education, and clinical care.*

# Contents

# Section One
## Management Strategies

# 1   Amblyopia Treatment

Amblyopia is poor vision caused by abnormal visual stimulation during early visual development. The abnormal visual stimulation disrupts neuro-development of visual centers in the brain. Abnormal stimulation can arise from a blurred retinal image, or strabismus with strong fixation preference for one eye and cortical suppression of the nondominant eye. Children under 8 years of age are capable of strong cortical suppression and hence can eliminate double vision. Children who alternate fixation and use either eye will alternate suppression and do not develop amblyopia. The **vertical prism induced tropia test** can be used to determine fixation preference and diagnose unilateral amblyopia in preverbal children with straight eyes or small angle strabismus.[1] This test is performed by placing a vertically oriented 10 PD prism over one eye, either base down or base up. The vertical prism induces a hypertropia allowing evaluation of fixation preference. Strong fixation preference for one eye is indicative of amblyopia.[2] Amblyopia can be bilateral in children with bilateral blurred retinal images (e.g., bilateral congenital cataracts, or bilateral high hypermetropia >+5.00 sphere).

Vision is the foremost priority in ophthalmology so strabismic children with amblyopia should have the amblyopia treated prior to strabismus surgery. After strabismus surgery the parents often assume that all is well, and will default follow up appointments. Thus our best chance for treating amblyopia is before strabismus surgery. An exception to this rule is amblyopia associated with large angle esotropia, with the amblyopic eye fixed in adduction (**strabismus fixus**) so the visual axis is occluded. Part of the amblyopia treatment is to operate on the amblyopic eye to bring it into primary position, to clear the visual axis and allow occlusion therapy.

Amblyopia therapy works best when initiated in young children under 3 years of age, however, even older children up to 8 to 9 years of age, can show visual acuity improvement with diligent amblyopia therapy. It is also important to monitor children after strabismus surgery for the development of amblyopia until the ages of 8 to 9 years. The two basic strategies to treat amblyopia are:

1. Provide a clear retinal image.
2. Correct ocular dominance.

## Clear Retinal Image

The first goal of amblyopia therapy is to ensure the presence of a clear retinal image. A careful **cycloplegic refraction** is required for all children with amblyopia and strabismus. Topical cyclopentolate 1% with tropicamide

1% given twice can achieve adequate cycloplegia for most patients. Patients with densely pigmented irides may require multiple drops, or even atropine 1% given twice a day for three days if retinoscopy shows variable readings.

Table 1.1 lists refractive errors that are potentially amblyogenic and need correction. Prescribing spectacles for patients with accommodative esotropia is covered in Chapter 4. Patients with straight eyes and anisometropic amblyopia usually have some degree of peripheral fusion. These patients often show significant visual acuity improvement with optical correction alone, even without occlusion therapy. As a rule, give the full hypermetropic correction to the amblyopic eye because amblyopic eyes do not

TABLE 1.1. When is a refractive error amblyogenic?

| Type of Amblyopia | Refractive Error Requiring Correction |
|---|---|
| Hypermetropic anisometropia | >+1.50 D of anisometropia |
| Myopic anisometropia | >−4.00 D of anisometropia |
| Astigmatic anisometropia | >+1.50 D anisometropia |
| Bilateral hypermetropia | >+5.00 D OU |
| Bilateral astigmatism | >+2.50 D OU |

These are only suggestions for prescribing spectacles in children, based on the cycloplegic refraction. Decisions on whether or not to treat a specific refractive error should be based on the whole clinical picture including visual acuity when attainable.

## Example 1.1.  Anisometropic Amblyopia

3-year old

VA:    OD 20/25
       OS 20/100

Cycloplegic refraction:    OD +1.00 sphere
                           OS +3.50 sphere

Stereo acuity without correction: 400 seconds arc (1/3 animals Titmus test)
Alignment: Orthotropia for distance and near

**Diagnosis:** Anisometropic Amblyopia OS with good binocular function

**Treatment:** Prescribe spectacles:
          OD + 0.50 sphere
          OS + 3.25 sphere

Note that the plus was slightly reduced (OD more than OS) to facilitate tolerance for spectacle use. Patient to return every 4 weeks to monitor visual acuity improvement. If improvement plateaus, then start part-time occlusion of the right eye 3 to 5 hours a day.

> ## Example 1.2.  Bilateral Hypermetropic Amblyopia
>
> 5-year old
>
> VA: 20/200 OU
>
> Cycloplegic refraction: +8.00 sphere OU
> Alignment: Orthotropia for distance and near
>
> **Treatment:** Prescribe spectacles with the full plus +8.00 sphere OU
> Note that patients with bilateral high hypermetropic amblyopia will not fully accommodate so they need their full plus correction to provide a clear retinal image. These patients usually have straight eyes and do not typically have accommodative esotropia as they hypoaccommodate.

fully accommodate. If the good eye is mildly hyperopic (+0.75 to +1.50 sphere) it is advisable not to give the full plus to the good eye as this will blur the vision and the child may not wear the spectacles (see Example 1.1). The key is that the spectacles must be worn full time—even in the bath tub or swimming pool!

Patients with bilateral high hypermetropia (>+5.00 sphere) will have bilateral amblyopia. These patients are so hypermetropic that they do not fully accommodate and they do not typically develop accommodative esotropia. They require full hypermetropic correction to provide a clear retinal image and treat the amblyopia (see Example 1.2).

## Correct Ocular Dominance

Patients with unilateral amblyopia will have strong dominance for the "good eye" and will suppress the amblyopic eye. Part of the strategy to treat amblyopia is to stimulate the amblyopic eye by forcing fixation to the amblyopic eye. There are two ways to switch fixation to the amblyopic eye: 1) occlude the dominant eye, and 2) blur the vision of the dominant eye (penalization).

### Occlusion Therapy

Occlusion therapy consists of patching the sound eye to force fixation to the amblyopic eye. For patients with binocular fusion and amblyopia (e.g., intermittent esotropia and anisometropic amblyopia), part time occlusion therapy is preferred over full time in order to maintain binocular fusion. If the child has a constant esotropia and no fusion (e.g., congenital esotropia) then full time occlusion can be done. Follow-up visits for full time occlusion therapy should be scheduled at intervals of 1 week per year of the child's age. For example, a 2-year old should be checked every 2 weeks to examine the good eye for occlusion induced amblyopia in addition to monitoring visual improvement of the amblyopic eye. In children less than 1 year of age, part time occlusion, half of the waking hours, is suggested to avoid the complication of occlusion amblyopia of the good eye.

*Penalization Therapy*

Penalization works by blurring the image of the sound eye to force fixation to the amblyopic eye. Blurring of the sound eye can be accomplished by adhesive tape on the spectacle lens, a blurring optical lens, or by atropine drops if the "good eye" is hypermetropic. Atropine penalization consists of instilling one drop of atropine 1% in the sound eye each day and removing the optical correction of the sound eye, while full optical correction is given to the amblyopic eye. If the cycloplegia of the good eye blurs the vision enough to switch fixation to the amblyopic eye then atropine penalization will usually improve vision.[3] The vertical prism induced tropia test can be used to determine which eye is fixating. The "good eye" has to be hypermetropic (at least +2.00 sphere) in order for atropine cycloplegia to blur the vision enough to force fixation to the amblyopic eye at least for near targets (see Example 1.3). Atropine has been reported to have a beneficial effect from the age of three years to seven years old and with an acuity of 20/40 to 20/100.[4] When atropine penalization works, it can provide strong anti-suppression therapy which may result in reverse amblyopia and loss of vision of the sound eye. To avoid reverse amblyopia, patients should be followed closely at intervals of one week per year of the patient's age not to exceed 3 weeks. Stop penalization if visual acuity in the "good eye" decreases.

---

### Example 1.3. Penalization (see Figure 1.1)

5-year old, patching failure

VA:  OD 20/200
     OS 20/30

Cycloplegic refraction:  OD +5.50 sphere
                         OS +3.00 sphere

Stereo acuity without correction: 3000 seconds arc (Positive fly Titmus test)
Alignment: Orthotropia for distance and near

**Diagnosis:** Dense amblyopia, patching failure

**Treatment:** Optical correction right eye—no correction left eye and atropine drops once a day:  OD + 5.50 sphere
                         OS plano + Atropine 1% every day

Note: The goal is to blur the vision of the "good eye" (left eye) with atropine and no optical correction in order to switch fixation to the amblyopic eye (right eye) that has full optical correction. If atropine penalization induces a switch in fixation to the amblyopic eye then vision will improve. If the patient continues to fixate with the atropinized good eye, then vision in the amblyopic eye will not improve. In these cases patching plus atropine penalization may be effective. Note that for atropine penalization to work the "good eye" must be significantly hypermetropic (>+2.00 sphere).

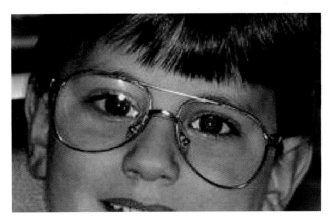

**Figure 1.1.** Atropine penalization left eye. Left eye is treated with atropine 1% every day and removal of optical correction. Note that the left pupil is dilated and the spectacle lens has been removed.

## End Point for Amblyopia Treatment

Amblyopia treatment is usually continued until vision in the amblyopic eye improves to within 1 or 2 Snellen lines of the sound eye. After improvement is achieved maintenance therapy, consisting of part time occlusion (1 to 2 hours a day) of the sound eye, may be necessary until the patient is 7 to 8 years old. Patients with anisometropic amblyopia and binocular fusion tend to maintain their vision after being treated, even without maintenance occlusion therapy, as long as optical correction is continued.

## References

1. Wright KW, Walonker F, Edelman P. 10-Diopter fixation test for amblyopia. Arch Ophthalmol 1981;99:1242–1246.
2. Wright KW, Edelman PM, Walonker F, Yiu S. Reliability of fixation preference testing in diagnosing amblyopia. Arch Ophthalmol 1986;104:549–553.
3. Wright KW, Guyton DL. A test for predicting the effectiveness of penalization on amblyopia. In: Henkind P, ed. Acta: XXIV International Congress of Ophthalmology. Philadelphia: JB Lippincott,1983;896–901.
4 Pediatric Eye Disease Investigator Group. The course of moderate amblyopia treated with atropine in children: experience of the amblyopia treatment study. Am J Ophthalmol 2003;136:630–639.

# 2 Principles of Strabismus Surgery

## Planning for Success

Prior to strabismus surgery an important and seemingly obvious question should be asked, "Why are we operating?" Is our treatment goal to establish binocular fusion, eliminate diplopia, expand the field of binocular vision, correct a compensatory head posture, or to simply improve cosmetic appearance? Establishing the goals prior to surgery helps us clarify indications for surgery, and formulate a logical treatment plan. A plan that is best for the patient should be made; not just a plan that is best for correcting the angle of deviation.

The indications for surgery should be based on the patient's needs: either binocular function or cosmetic appearance (Table 2.1). Urgent surgery is indicated to reestablish binocular fusion in a child with an esophoria that has recently broken down to a tropia. The family should be told that surgery is indicated to regain binocular fusion and not just to improve the cosmetic appearance. In contrast, surgery for a long-standing sensory esotropia secondary to a blind eye is cosmetic, as there is virtually no potential for binocular fusion. In this case the indication for surgery should be based on the cosmetic desires of the patient. In some cases it may be difficult, or even impossible to determine the binocular potential. For example, an older child with equal vision and a history of esotropia since infancy may or may not have binocular fusion potential. In these cases, I tend to give the patient the benefit of doubt, and treat the patient as if they have fusion potential.

Understanding the functional goal also helps direct the surgical plan. Esotropic patients with fusion potential generally require large amounts of surgery, more than the standard surgical numbers (see Chapter 4). A plan based on standard surgery in these patients routinely results in undercorrection. Esotropic patients without binocular fusion potential, however, are ill served by planning for "more" surgery as a consecutive exotropia will inevitably increase over time and an exotropia is a poor cosmetic outcome. In these cases without fusion potential, it is better to do less surgery, as a small residual esotropia is more stable and has a better appearance than a consecutive exotropia. Consideration of the functional outcome also influences the selection of the type of surgery. Monocular recession-resection surgery produces incomitance which is not optimal in a fusing patient, as incomitance can cause diplopia in eccentric positions of gaze. Monocular surgery on the blind eye is, however, the procedure of choice for sensory strabismus to protect the only seeing good eye. These are but a few examples that demonstrate the importance of considering the potential for

**TABLE 2.1.** Indications for Strabismus Surgery

***Binocular Functional***
   Establish Binocular Fusion
     1. Early surgery infantile esotropia
     2. Partially accommodative esotropia
     3. Decompensated intermittent exotropia
   Binocular Diplopia
     1. Acquired incomitant strabismus (restriction or paresis)
     2. Acquired comitant strabismus
     3. Postoperative anomalous retinal correspondence—paradoxical diplopia
   Binocular Field
     1. Expand binocular visual field
     2. Correct face turn or head tilt (associated with nystagmus or incomitant strabismus)
***Cosmetic Appearance***
   1. Sensory strabismus (associated with unilateral poor vision or dense amblyopia)
   2. Long-standing infantile strabismus (late surgery for congenital esotropia)
   3. Lid fissure changes (Duane's syndrome III co-contraction)

**TABLE 2.2.** Signs of Binocular Fusion Potential

1. Intermittent strabismus
2. Acquired strabismus (old photographs showing straight eyes)
3. Binocular fusion or stereo acuity after neutralizing the deviation with prisms or amblyoscope
4. Infant <2 years old and equal vision
5. Incomitant strabismus with compensatory face posturing

binocular fusion when planning strabismus surgery. Table 2.2 lists some important signs that indicate the potential for binocular fusion.

Prior to surgery it is helpful to establish a specific strabismus diagnosis. In most cases the strabismus can be classified into a type, such as partially accommodative esotropia, intermittent exotropia, Duane's syndrome—esotropia type 1, congenital superior oblique palsy, or Brown's syndrome. At times, it may be difficult to determine the exact etiology of the strabismus. In these cases an MRI of the head and orbit may be indicated. If after a complete evaluation the cause is unknown, then it is appropriate to operate for the strabismus pattern taking into account the ductions, versions, and the presence of incomitance.

## Paradoxical Diplopia

Planning strabismus surgery for adult patients with childhood strabismus offers a special challenge as they may have **anomalous retinal correspondence (ARC)** and develop postoperative *paradoxical diplopia*. ARC is a sensory adaptation where the true fovea is suppressed and an eccentric retinal point corresponding to the deviation is considered the center of vision (pseudofovea). When the strabismus is corrected the pseudofovea is now out of alignment, so the patient will see double even though the eyes appear in anatomical alignment. Paradoxical diplopia is usually not as bothersome as diplopia associated with normal retinal correspondence and patients know which is the "real" image. In most cases paradoxical diplopia will resolve spontaneously over several days to months. Rarely, however, patients may have persistent diplopia requiring prisms, or even additional strabismus surgery, to reverse the correction and re-create the original strabismus.

An important test to predict if an adult is at risk for postoperative diplopia is the **prism neutralization test**. Neutralize the deviation with a prism and ask the patient if they see double. Test for diplopia in free view, then repeat prism neutralization with a red filter over one eye and use a hand light as a fixation target. If the patient sees double with the deviation neutralized the patient should be advised that they will probably see double after surgery. If the patient does not experience bothersome diplopia with prism neutralization, one can operate to correct the full deviation. Paradoxical diplopia is not as bothersome as normal correspondence diplopia. Another approach is to use prism neutralization to find the largest angle of correction that avoids diplopia, and use that as the target angle even though it will result in an undercorrection. It is a good rule to inform all adult patients that postoperative diplopia is a possibility.

## How Does Strabismus Surgery Work?

Strabismus surgery corrects ocular misalignment by slackening a muscle (i.e., recession), by tightening a muscle (i.e., resection), or by changing the insertion site of the muscle, thus changing the direction of pull or vector of force (i.e., transposition).

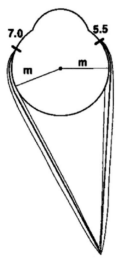

**FIGURE 2.1.** Diagram of the horizontal rectus muscles showing the relationship of the moment arm *(m)* to the muscle axis and center of rotation. The moment arm intersects the center of rotation and is perpendicular to the muscle axis. The longer the moment arm and the stronger the muscle force, the greater the rotational force.

## LENGTH TENSION CURVE

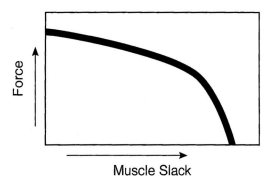

FIGURE 2.2. Starling's length-tension curve: The relationship of a muscle's force is proportional to the tension on the muscle. More tension on a muscle will increase muscle force, and slackening a muscle will reduce its force. Note the relationship is not linear, but exponential. Towards the end of the curve a small degree of slackening produces a disproportionately large amount of muscle weakening.

When a muscle contracts it produces a force that rotates the globe in a particular direction (muscle action) with a certain rotational force. **Rotational force** that moves an eye is directly proportional to the length of the moment arm (m) and the force of the muscle contraction (F).

$$\text{Rotational Force} = m \times F$$

where, $m$ = moment arm and $F$ = muscle force.

## Muscle Recession

A muscle recession moves the muscle insertion to a new location closer to the muscle's origin creating muscle slack. Muscle slack created by a recession reduces muscle strength as per Starling's length tension curve. The initial slackening of muscle fibers is taken up by fiber reorganization but there is probably a persistent change in both the recessed muscle and the antagonist. Surgical charts on the amount of recession for a specific deviation reflect the exponential character of the length tension curve. For example, each 0.5 mm of a bilateral medial rectus recession will correct approximately 5 prism diopters (PD) of esotropia up to a recession of 5.5 mm. However, after 5.5 mm of recession, each additional 0.5 mm of recession results in 10 PD of correction. Clinically, this is important, as we must be extremely careful when measuring large recessions because relatively small errors in measurement will result in large errors in eye alignment. An inadvertent over recession of only 1.0 mm on a planned 6.0 mm bilateral medial rectus recession could result in a 20 PD overcorrection.

A unilateral rectus muscle recession will induce incomitance, as rectus muscle recessions have more of an effect in the field of action of the muscle. Note that when the eye rotates towards the recessed muscle *(right drawing)*, the moment arm shortens and muscle slack increases. This results in progressive weakening of the rotational force as the eye turns towards the recessed muscle. In contrast, on eye rotation away from the recessed

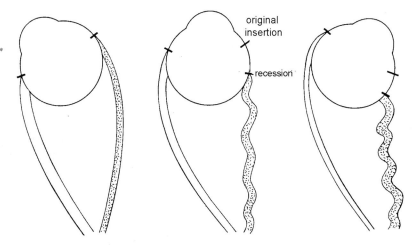

**FIGURE 2.3.** Drawing shows a rectus muscle recession. Note that in primary position (center drawing) the length of the moment arm remains unchanged and is equal to the radius. Thus, the effect of a standard rectus muscle recession on a strabismus in primary position is not due to a change in leverage, but is based on the amount of muscle slack created. This is of practical importance because when measuring a recession, measure from the muscle insertion to quantify the amount of slack produced.

muscle *(left drawing)*, the moment arm is at full length, and muscle slack is reduced. In addition, on eye rotation away from the recessed muscle, the recessed muscle is inhibited (Sherrington's law of agonist and antagonist) so the effect of the recession is minimal (Examples 2.1 and 2.2). For example, a right medial rectus recession will produce an exoshift in primary position and a larger exoshift in left gaze with very little exoshift in right gaze. A unilateral or asymmetric recession, therefore, will induce incomitance, whereas bilateral symmetrical recessions will produce a comitant result. Procedures that induce incomitance are used to treat incomitant strabismus.

---

*Example 2.1.  How would you best correct this esotropia with a recession? (Forced ductions are negative)*

| Right gaze | Primary position | Left gaze |
|------------|------------------|-----------|
| ET 25 PD   | ET 15 PD         | ET 5 PD   |

Answer: Recess the Left medial rectus muscle.

Note that a left medial rectus muscle recession would have more of an effect in right gaze where the deviation is maximum. A right medial rectus muscle recession would induce an exotropia in left gaze and leave a residual esotropia in right gaze if the esotropia in primary position is corrected.

*Example 2.2.  How would you best correct this right hypertropia with a recession? (Forced ductions are negative)*

Up gaze RHT 5 PD

Primary position RHT 10 PD

Down gaze RHT 15 PD

Answer: Recess the Left inferior rectus muscle.

Note that a left inferior rectus muscle recession would have more of an effect in down gaze where the deviation is maximum. A right superior rectus recession would have more of an effect in up gaze resulting in a left hypertropia in up gaze (overcorrection), and leave a residual right hypertropia in down gaze if the right hypertropia in primary position is corrected.

Recessions are routinely performed on rectus muscles, but can also be performed on oblique muscles. Inferior oblique muscle recession is a popular procedure for weakening the inferior oblique muscle and is described in more detail in Chapter 17. Recession of the superior oblique tendon can weaken the superior oblique muscle but moving the broad insertion of the superior oblique tendon anterior and nasal can produce limitation of depression postoperatively. A more controlled method of slackening the tendon is a tendon lengthening procedure, the "Wright silicone tendon expander" (see Chapter 19).

## Muscle Tightening Procedures (Resection, Tuck, and Plication)

Rectus muscle tightening procedures include resections, tucks, and plications. These procedures tighten by shortening the muscle. Increased muscle tension will result in muscle fiber hypertrophy and this has been described as a temporary effect after muscle resection in the animal model. After a few weeks the muscle fiber diameter returned to baseline.[1] Thus muscle tightening procedures have a relatively small effect on the length tension curve and no effect on the moment arm. For the most part, muscle tightening procedures correct strabismus by creating a tether, or a leash, not by increasing muscle function. Often a resection is touted as a muscle strengthening procedure, but in reality removing a section of the muscle tightens the muscle but does not improve muscle strength. Clinically, a resection produces incomitance as the tightened muscle restricts rotation away from the resected muscle (Figure 2.4). For example, a medial rectus resection limits abduction (Example 2.3). It should be noted that tightening both medial rectus muscles restricts divergence and creates an esoshift which is greater in the distance than near. Tightening the medial rectus muscles does not improve convergence and is not effective in correcting convergence insufficiency.

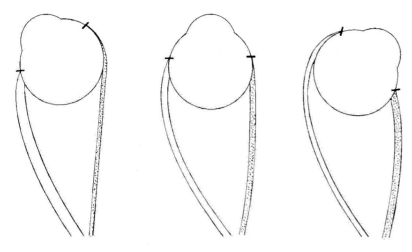

**FIGURE 2.4.** The effect of a rectus muscle tightening procedure, such as a resection. Note that the tightened muscle (the shaded muscle) causes restriction and limits eye rotation away from the tight muscle.

---

*Example 2.3.  How would you best correct this esotropia with a resection?*

| Right gaze | Primary position | Left gaze |
|---|---|---|
| ET 25 PD | ET 15 PD | ET 5 PD |

Answer: Resect the Left lateral rectus muscle.

Note that a left lateral rectus muscle resection would restrict adduction thus inducing an exoshift in right gaze and correcting the esotropia that increases in right gaze. A right lateral rectus muscle resection would correct the esotropia in primary position but would induce an exotropia in left gaze and leave a residual esotropia in right gaze.

---

*Resection*

A muscle **resection** consists of tightening a muscle by excising part of the muscle and reattaching the shortened muscle at its original insertion site (Chapter 14). Resections are usually performed on rectus muscles, not the oblique muscles.

*Tuck*

Another technique to tighten or shorten a muscle is the muscle **tuck**. A tuck is a procedure that shortens the muscle by folding the muscle and suturing the folded muscle to muscle. The tendon tuck of rectus muscles has, for the most part, fallen out of favor partially because the muscle to muscle suturing did not hold well. The major muscle fibers are longitudinal and the transverse connective tissue fibers are weak. Muscle to muscle tucks pull through the weak transverse muscle fibers and loose their effect over time. An exception are tucks on the superior oblique tendon as this is performed on the tendon—not muscle.

*Plication*

The author has developed the rectus muscle plication procedure.[2] The plication shortens the muscle by securing the muscle posterior to the insertion (as in a resection or tuck) then securing the sutures to sclera to shorten the muscle. The rectus plication tightens the rectus muscle while preserving the anterior ciliary circulation. The muscle to sclera plication provides a stable result as the muscle is anchored to the sclera. The procedure is described in Chapter 14. A superior oblique tendon plication is used for some cases of superior oblique palsy (Chapter 18).

## Recession and Resection

Resections (and Wright plication) can be combined with recessions of the same eye, and this is called a **recession–resection**, or an "**R & R**" procedure. The effect of the recession and resection is additive in regards to limiting eye rotation. The recession reduces rotational force towards the recessed muscle while the resection restricts rotation away from the resected muscle. Thus, the recession–resection procedure causes significant incomitance. For example, a recession of the left lateral rectus muscle and resection of the left medial rectus muscle to treat a comitant exotropia will correct the exotropia in primary position, but would create an esotropia in left gaze. This is because the left eye would have limitation of abduction as compared to the normal adduction of the unoperated right eye. Limited rotations after an R & R procedure usually improve over several months to years, but some residual incomitance often persists. Since the R & R procedure induces incomitance, it is best used to treat incomitant strabismus. Monocular R & R is also the procedure of choice for the treatment of sensory strabismus so surgery is performed only on the blind eye.

## Faden

Faden means suture in German. The faden procedure consists of a suture placed through a rectus muscle securing the muscle to posterior sclera, usually 12 mm to 14 mm posterior to the muscle insertion. This procedure reduces rotational force by shortening the moment arm when the eye rotates toward the muscle with the faden. It has minimal effect in primary position, but progressively reduces the rotational force as the eye rotates towards the operated muscle. The faden has a relatively weak effect so it is almost always used in conjunction with a muscle recession (Chapter 20). It is most effective on the medial rectus muscle as the medial rectus muscle has the shortest arc of contact.

## Muscle Transposition

Transposition surgery is based on changing the location of the muscle insertion so the muscle pulls the eye in a direction different than the normal action of the muscle (i.e., changes the vector of force). Transposition surgeries can be used to treat a rectus muscle paresis (Chapter 16), A and V patterns (Chapter 15), small vertical tropias (Chapter 15), and torsion (Chapter 15). A right lateral rectus palsy results in an esotropia with limited abduction. The lack of lateral force can be treated by transposing all or part of the superior rectus and inferior rectus muscles laterally to the lateral rectus insertion (Chapter 16). Since the vertical muscles do not contract on abduction, the amount of abduction would depend on the elasticity of the transposed muscles, not on the active contraction of the muscles.

Vertical transposition of horizontal rectus muscle insertions can correct small vertical deviations (Chapter 15). A small right hypertropia, for example, can be corrected by infraplacement of the right medial and lateral rectus muscles. Transposing the horizontal rectus muscles inferiorly towards the inferior rectus muscle changes the function of the horizontal recti to act to pull the eye down, thus correcting the hypertropia.

Transposition of the inferior oblique muscle insertion anterior to the equator is an excellent way to treat inferior oblique overaction. The author developed the graded anteriorization to quantify the amount of inferior oblique muscle weakening.[3] By moving the insertion anteriorly, the inferior oblique muscle becomes more of a depressor and less of an elevator. The more anterior the insertion, the more the weakening effect (Chapter 17).

## References

1. Christiansen S et al. Fiber hypertrophy in rat extraocular muscle following lateral rectus resection. J Pediatr Ophthalmol Strabismus 1988;25(4):167–171.
2. Wright KW, Lanier, AB. Effect of a modified rectus tuck on anterior segment circulation in monkeys. J Pediatr Ophthalmol Strabismus 1991;28:77–81.
3. Guemes A, Wright KW. Effect of graded anterior transposition of the inferior oblique muscle on versions and vertical deviation in primary position. J AAPOS 1998;2:201–206.

# 3  Infantile Esotropia

An esotropia (ET) presenting during the first 6 months of life is termed infantile esotropia. There are various presentations of infantile esotropia with the following forms being the most common: small angle neonatal esotropia, congenital esotropia, Ciancia's syndrome, and accommodative infantile esotropia. Normal newborn infants typically have a small exotropia (>70% of normal neonates) that usually resolves by 4 to 6 months of age. Infantile esotropia, on the other hand, is rare, and usually does not resolve spontaneously.

## Small Angle Neonatal Esotropia

### Clinical Features

- ET 15 to 35 PD, variable angle
- Onset birth to 2 months of age
- Approximately 30% will resolve spontaneously by 6 months of age

### Etiology

Unknown etiology

### Clinical Evaluation

**Amblyopia:** Unusual as the deviation is often intermittent and there is some binocular fusion. Unless strong fixation preference is present, do not treat with patching, as this could break down weak fusion. Treat amblyopia by patching the dominant eye 2 to 4 hours a day until the patient holds fixation well with the non-dominant eye. Follow up every 1 to 2 weeks to test for change in fixation preference. A week or two of patching can reverse fixation preference in these young infants.

**Cycloplegic Refraction:** Use cyclopentolate 1% one or two doses, 5 minutes apart. Refract 30 minutes after the last dose.

**Complete Ocular Examination:** A complete ocular examination including a dilated retinal exam is important to rule out a sensory esotropia. Sensory esotropia can be caused by an infantile cataract, retinoblastoma, optic nerve hypoplasia, or any other cause of infantile visual loss.

*Management*

The Congenital Esotropia Observational Study (CEOS) sponsored by the National Institute of Health has shown that infants with a small angle (≤35 PD), variable, or intermittent esotropia have a high rate of spontaneous resolution as approximately one third will resolve by 6 months of age.[1] These infants should have a cycloplegic refraction and if hypermetropic of +3.00 sphere or more, give spectacles with the full correction (see Infantile Accommodative Esotropia later in this Chapter). If not significantly hypermetropic, observe until the infant is 6 to 9 months old for spontaneous resolution. Some patients will show an increasing esotropia and they should be considered for early surgery if the deviation becomes constant and is ≥40 PD seen on at least two consecutive exams (see congenital esotropia below).

**Premature Infants** will frequently have a small variable esotropia. There is not much in the literature to guide us in these cases. It is probably best to watch these patients for several months for spontaneous resolution. Consider surgery at 9 to 12 months of corrected age if a constant esotropia >15 to 20 PD persists, and the child is not a significant anesthesia risk.

**Surgical Procedure:** Surgery is based on the near deviation as this is the most reliable measurement in these young children. Bilateral medial rectus (MR) recessions are preferred because the deviation is usually comitant. If there is unilateral vision loss then a monocular recession–tightening procedure is performed on the poor seeing eye.

# Congenital Esotropia

*Clinical Features*

- Large angle constant esotropia (≥40 PD)
- Onset from birth to 6 months of age
- Spontaneous resolution is rare
- Amblyopia common (50%)
- Associated motor phenomena *(usually present after 2 years of age)*
  1. Inferior Oblique Overaction (IOOA) (60%)
  2. Dissociated Vertical Deviation (DVD) (40%)
  3. Latent nystagmus (40%)

**Smooth Pursuit Asymmetry/Optokinetic Nystagmus Asymmetry:** Normal children and adults have precise and symmetrical smooth pursuit for following an object moving slowly from side to side. Infants, however, have smooth pursuit asymmetry with a deficiency in nasal to temporal smooth pursuit, as compared to pursuit following an object moving in a temporal to nasal direction. This asymmetry is only demonstrated during monocular viewing. Smooth pursuit asymmetry is a manifestation of visual motor immaturity and naturally resolves as motor fusion develops by 4 to 6 months of age. Patients with disorders that disrupt binocular visual development such as congenital esotropia, or unilateral congenital cataract retain smooth pursuit asymmetry throughout life, despite surgery.[2] Thus, the presence of smooth pursuit asymmetry in older children and adults with esotropia is a sign of neonatal onset with early disruption of binocular visual development.

*Etiology*

Unknown etiology

*Preoperative Evaluation*

**Ductions:** Mild (−1) limitation of abduction is common and does not indicate a lateral rectus paresis. Try the doll's head maneuver or spinning the child (vestibular stimulation) to elicit full abduction. Intact abduction saccadic eye movements in the face of mild limitation of abduction indicates good lateral rectus function and a tight medial rectus muscle.

**Differential Diagnosis of Infantile ET with Limited Abduction:** This list is in order of decreasing incidence.

- Ciancia's syndrome (tight medial rectus muscles—see below)
- Duane's syndrome
- Congenital fibrosis syndrome
- Congenital sixth nerve palsy (very rare—usually transient, resolving by 4 months of age)
- Infantile myasthenia gravis

**Versions:** Check for inferior oblique overaction and V-pattern.

**Amblyopia:** Check fixation preference—strong preference for one eye indicates amblyopia.

**Measure Deviation:** Prism alternate cover is best, but use Krimsky testing for verification, or if prism cover testing is unobtainable. Surgery is usually based on the near deviation as this is the most reliable in infants. When possible, measure the distance and near deviation.

**Cycloplegic Refraction:** Use cyclopentolate 1% one or two doses, 5 minutes apart. Refract 30 minutes after the last dose.

*Management*

In general, congenital esotropia is a surgical disease and requires strabismus surgery. If the cycloplegic refraction shows ≥+3.00 sphere, then prescribe the full hypermetropic correction. If after prescribing the full hypermetropic correction an esotropia of >10 to 15 PD persists, then surgery is required (see infantile accommodative esotropia below).

**Amblyopia:** Treat amblyopia before surgery, by patching the dominant eye 4 to 6 hours per day until the patient holds fixation well with the nondominant eye. Follow up every 1 to 2 weeks, to test for change in fixation preference. A week or two of patching can reverse fixation preference in these young infants Patients may *cross-fixate*, fixing with the right eye for objects in the left visual field and with the left eye for objects in the right visual field. Unless strong fixation preference is present, cross-fixation usually indicates absence of significant amblyopia.

**Timing of Surgery for Congenital ET:** Most references recommend that surgery for congenital esotropia be performed between 6 months and 1 year of age in order to achieve peripheral fusion and low grade stereo acuity. This author reported experience with very early surgery showing that surgical correction between 3 and 4 months of age can result in high grade stereo acuity.[3] Early surgery should be considered if there is constant large angle esotropia (≥40 PD) with the angle stable or increasing on at least two examinations, two or more weeks apart. CEOS showed that spontaneous resolution was rare (<4%) if these parameters were met.[4] Intermittent small angle esotropia, on the other hand, will resolve in approximately one third of cases, so in these patients it is better to wait until at least 6 months of age before considering surgery.

**Surgical Procedure:** The procedure of choice is bilateral medial rectus (MR) muscle recessions using the near deviation as the target angle (use surgical chart in appendix for specific numbers). The standard surgical chart numbers are designed to give infants with infantile esotropia a slight immediate overcorrection, which is desirable as convergence will pull the eyes straight (see Surgical Goals later in this chapter). In older patients and adults with long-standing congenital esotropia the chart numbers may give a slight undercorrection. This is desirable as they usually have poor fusion potential and tend to drift to exotropia over time. Thus the surgical chart numbers can be used for all ages as they tend to self adjust for age. Patients with irreversible dense amblyopia should have monocular surgery on the amblyopic eye (recession-tightening procedure) to protect the "good eye."

---

## Example 3.1.  Clinical Example: Congenital ET (see Figure 3.1)

- 5-month old, constant large esotropia since first few weeks of life.
- Strong fixation preference OD
- Ductions—trace limitation to abduction, versions—no oblique dysfunction
- Full abduction and good saccade to vestibular stimulation (doll's head maneuver).
- Cycloplegic refraction
  OD +1.75 sphere
  OS +2.00 sphere

Nsc: ET 60 PD by alternate cover test and Krimsky prism test
Dsc: ET 50 PD by estimation
(D = distance, N = near, sc = without correction)

**Diagnosis:** Congenital esotropia, strabismic amblyopia left eye, slightly limited abduction probably secondary to tight medial rectus muscles, but not a sixth nerve paresis because there is a good abduction saccade.

**Preoperative Treatment:** Patch right eye 6 hours a day and follow every week until equal fixation preference is achieved, indicating that amblyopia has improved. At 5 months of age only one or two weeks of patching are usually needed to improve the amblyopia.

**Surgery:** Bilateral medial rectus muscle recessions 6.5 mm for target angle ET 60 PD (see Appendix I on Surgical Numbers). Note: Do not prescribe spectacles preoperatively, however, if there is a small residual esotropia after surgery try prescribing the full hypermetropic correction.

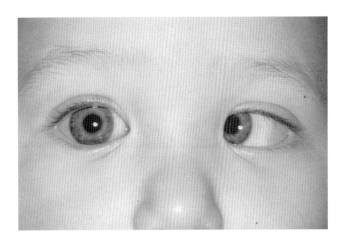

**FIGURE 3.1.** A 5-month old with congenital esotropia.

**Surgical Goals:** The immediate postoperative goal is a small exotropia (5 to 10 PD) for infants with possible fusion potential. A small exotropia is "good" as we naturally have strong innate fusional convergence (>30 PD), so a small exotropia can be fused. A small esotropia, on the other hand, is difficult to fuse, as our divergence amplitudes are weak (approximately 8 PD).

Dr. Marshall Parks, during his studies on monofixation syndrome and peripheral fusion, found that in order to develop binocular fusion the eyes must be within 8 to 10 PD of orthotropia. The goal of surgery is to align the eyes early during infancy to within 8 to 10 PD, to stimulate the development of binocular fusion. The closer the alignment to orthotropia, the better the sensory outcome. An esotropia larger than 8 to 10 PD will not allow binocular fusion (not even peripheral fusion). A residual esotropia larger than 10 PD should be considered for further treatment (see next section below). Patients with a poor prognosis for binocular fusion (e.g., dense irreversible amblyopia, or older patients (>2 years old) with uncorrected congenital esotropia) should be considered for surgery based on cosmetic indications.

**Residual Esotropia:** For a residual esotropia first repeat the cycloplegic refraction. If there is a small residual esotropia 10 to 20 PD try prescribing the full hypermetropic correction, even as little as +1.50 sphere, to correct the ET to within 10 PD. If, after prescribing the full hypermetropic correction, there is a residual ET >15 PD, then consider further surgery.

- If the primary surgery was a bilateral MR recession ≤5.0 mm then re-recess the medial recti OU. Recessing both medial recti an additional 2.5 mm usually corrects about 25 PD of esotropia.
- If primary bilateral MR recessions were >5.0 mm then resect both lateral recti (LR). Reduce the standard resection numbers by about 1.0 mm to 2.0 mm because you get more of an effect resecting against a previous large MR recession. Consecutive exotropia is a common occurrence after LR resections for a residual esotropia.

**Consecutive Exotropia:** An immediate small exodeviation (10 to 15 PD) is usually "good" as most will improve over several days to weeks because convergence amplitudes are strong. A consecutive exotropia >15 PD that does not improve after 2 to 3 months may be surgically corrected. Consider slipped medial rectus muscle or a stretched scar of medial rectus insertion if the consecutive exotropia is associated with even mild adduction deficit (see also Chapter 21).

- Full ductions—slipped medial rectus muscle has been ruled out, so perform bilateral LR recessions.
- Limited adduction—slipped muscle or stretched scar of the medial rectus muscle is suspected so first explore the medial rectus muscles and advance the muscle if it has slipped. Consider using a nonabsorbable suture for the reoperation to prevent recurrence of the stretched scar.

### Prognosis of Congenital ET

Motor alignment can be achieved in approximately 80% of surgical cases. If alignment to within 8 PD of orthotropia is achieved before 2 years of age, then approximately 60% to 80% will achieve some degree of peripheral fusion and gross stereopsis (monofixation syndrome). Only a few cases of high grade stereo acuity have been reported. Very early surgery, as young as 3 to 4 months of age, may increase the chances of achieving binocular fusion and high grade stereo acuity. If the eyes are aligned after 2 years of age, there is only a small chance of obtaining binocular fusion.

## Ciancia's Syndrome (Cross-Fixation Congenital Esotropia)

### Clinical Features

- Large angle congenital esotropia (>70 PD)
- Tight medial rectus muscles
- Restricted abduction
- Face turn with fixing eye in adduction
- Abduction nystagmus (end point nystagmus)

Ciancia's syndrome is simply a very large angle (>70 PD) congenital esotropia associated with tight medial rectus muscles. This causes limited abduction and keeps both eyes fixed in adduction. Because the eyes are fixed in adduction the patient cross-fixates. They adopt a face turn to the right to fixate with the right eye for objects in the left visual field, and a face turn to the left to fixate with the left eye for objects in the right visual field (Figure 3.2). End point nystagmus occurs on attempted abduction as the eye tries to abduct against the tight medial rectus muscle. There is no pathologic nystagmus, and no nystagmus with the fixing eye in adduction (resting position). Ciancia reported a high percentage of his congenital esotropia patients with this syndrome.[5]

### Etiology

Unknown etiology; may represent a form of congenital fibrosis isolated to the medial rectus muscles.

### Preoperative Evaluation

The examination is the same as for patients with congenital esotropia stated above. Since these patients have limited abduction it is important to

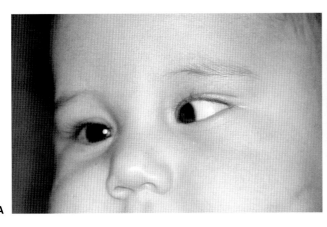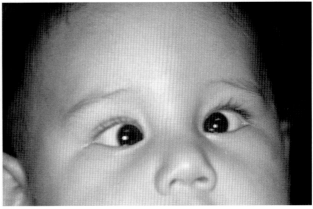

FIGURE 3.2. A 6-month old with Ciancia's syndrome type of congenital esotropia. The deviation measures at least 70 to 80 PD. The patient fixates in adduction because there is limited abduction caused by tight medial rectus muscles. Note the patient cross-fixes with the right eye fixing in adduction and a face turn to the right for viewing objects to the patient's left side (A). Likewise the left eye fixes in adduction and a face turn to the left for viewing objects to the patient's right side (B).

document the presence of abduction saccadic eye movements by doll's head maneuver or spinning the child. Intact abduction saccadic movements exclude sixth nerve palsy as a cause for limited abduction. Patients with Ciancia's syndrome will have intact abduction saccadic eye movements, but restriction to abduction because of tight medial rectus muscles.

**Amblyopia:** If vision is equal, patients will alternate fixation and adopt a face turn to the right to use their right eye for objects to the left, and face turn to the left to use their left eye for objects to the right. Patients with amblyopia will show strong fixation preference for one eye and face turn only to one side.

**Measuring the Deviation:** It is hard to accurately measure the full deviation because the fixing eye has difficulty coming to primary position. In general the deviation is underestimated. Fairly accurate measurements can be obtained by splitting the prism correction between the two eyes, then doing the alternate cover test. This requires a cooperative child and 3 hands so find a helper—good luck! Don't obsess over the measurements as maximal bilateral MR recessions are required.

*Management*

Ciancia's syndrome patients virtually always require surgery.

**Strabismus Fixus with Amblyopia:** Because of the large angle of strabismus some patients with Ciancia's syndrome will have one eye so turned in towards the nose that the nose actually blocks vision. This is called strabismus fixus and in infancy can lead to dense amblyopia. Usually patching does not work because the eye is fixed in adduction. In these cases if patching does not improve fixation, surgery should be performed (large bilateral MR recessions) to bring the eye to primary position and clear the visual axis. Patching of the dominant eye is then reinstituted.

**Surgical Procedure:** The treatment of Ciancia's syndrome is surgical. These patients require large bilateral medial rectus recessions (7.0 mm to 8 mm) as the medial recti are tight. The most common outcome is undercorrection because of residual tight medial rectus muscles. The Wright Grooved Hook (Yes, I have a financial interest) is very helpful for suturing these extremely tight muscles.

**Surgical Goals:** As in the case of congenital esotropia the goal is to align the eyes to within 8 to 10 PD, to allow stimulation of binocular visual development (see Congenital Esotropia earlier in this chapter).

**Residual Esotropia:** If there is a residual esotropia of >15 PD (a common result) consider further surgery. If there is residual limitation of abduction, and a residual face turn with the fixing eye in adduction, the medial rectus is probably still tight. In these cases forced ductions will show restriction to abduction. You have to re-recess the tight medial rectus muscle even if your primary surgery was a maximal medial rectus recession of 7.0 mm. This is not an easy surgery! A lateral rectus resection against a tight medial rectus will usually not work and will narrow the lid fissure.

An additional 2.5 mm to 3.5 mm bilateral medial rectus re-recession will correct approximately 20 to 30 PD of esotropia. Check the location of the medial rectus muscles. If the medial rectus is found at 7 mm or more behind the original insertion (12.5 mm from the limbus), then slightly reduce the re-recession. If the medial rectus is found less than 7 mm from the original insertion then increase the re-recession. The tightness of the medial rectus muscle should also influence the amount of re-recession. The tighter the muscle the greater the re-recession. Because the re-recession is far posterior and the muscle is tight, consider a limbal incision with the hang back technique. The Wright Grooved Hook is very helpful, almost mandatory, for suturing these tight posterior medial rectus muscles. Ok the Wright Grooved Hook again. Yes, I have a financial interest in the hook, but believe me, I still can't quit my day job!

**Consecutive Exotropia:** Overcorrection is unusual. An immediate small exodeviation (10 to 15 PD) is usually "good" as most will improve over several days to weeks because convergence amplitudes are strong. If an exotropia persists treat as stated above for congenital esotropia.

**Prognosis:** Patients with Ciancia's syndrome often end up with no discernable binocular fusion. When they do achieve fusion it is peripheral at best, and they rarely, if ever, achieve high grade stereo acuity. This poor sensory outcome may be due to the very high rate of residual esotropia.

## Infantile Accommodative Esotropia

*Clinical Features*

- Acquired esotropia, onset at 2 months to 1 year of age
- Hypermetropia > +2.50 sphere (usually +3.00 to +6.00 sphere)
- Variable deviation, often intermittent

*Etiology*

Patients with infantile accommodative esotropia are highly hypermetropic so they must accommodate an inordinate amount to see clearly. Linked with accommodation is convergence. When they overaccommodate they over converge, thus developing an esotropia. Dr. Gunter von Noorden of the United States would say somewhat jokingly that babies with type "A" personalities develop accommodative esotropia in infancy, while those with more of a laid back personality develop accommodative esotropia later in childhood. Why some hypermetropic patients do not develop esotropia is unknown but may relate to the AC/A ratio and divergence amplitudes.

*Clinical Evaluation*

**Cycloplegic refraction:** Use cyclopentolate 1% one or two doses, 5 minutes apart, and refract 30 minutes after the last dose. Repeat the cycloplegia if there are fluctuating readings on retinoscopy.

**Amblyopia:** First prescribe the full hypermetropic correction. After wearing the full correction for 4 weeks evaluate for fixation preference. If there is strong preference for one eye this indicates amblyopia. Treat amblyopia by patching the dominant eye 6 hours a day until the patient holds fixation well with the non-dominant eye.

**Measure Deviation:** Prism alternate cover testing is the most accurate method for measuring the deviation. Use an accommodative fixation target in order to reveal the full deviation. An accommodative target is a target with fine detail that requires full accommodation. Krimsky testing can also be used but alternate prism cover testing is preferred. Surgery is usually based on the near deviation.

*Management*

The goal is to establish straight eyes to stimulate the development of binocular fusion. If the eyes are within 8 to 10 PD of orthotropia with optical correction binocular fusion is possible and surgery is not indicated. These patients should be aggressively treated with early optical correction and early surgery if necessary. The late Dr. Marshall Parks, master of strabismus, considered recent onset accommodative esotropia as an ophthalmic urgency and would insist on seeing these patients the same day they called for an appointment.

**Spectacle Correction:** Prescribe the full hypermetropic correction immediately, even as early as 2 months of age. Spectacles must be worn full time. These patients with high hypermetropia will accept their full correction so do not wimp out—Give the full plus! Even if the spectacles slightly overcorrect the hypermetropia, say, by +0.50 sphere, mild myopia is trivial because an infant's world is up close. In the vast majority of cases the family will notice a significant improvement in the infant's visual behavior with the spectacles. My youngest son had accommodative esotropia with +5.50 sphere OU (Figure 3.3). I distinctly remember the immediate and dramatic improvement in visual behavior when he first dawned his

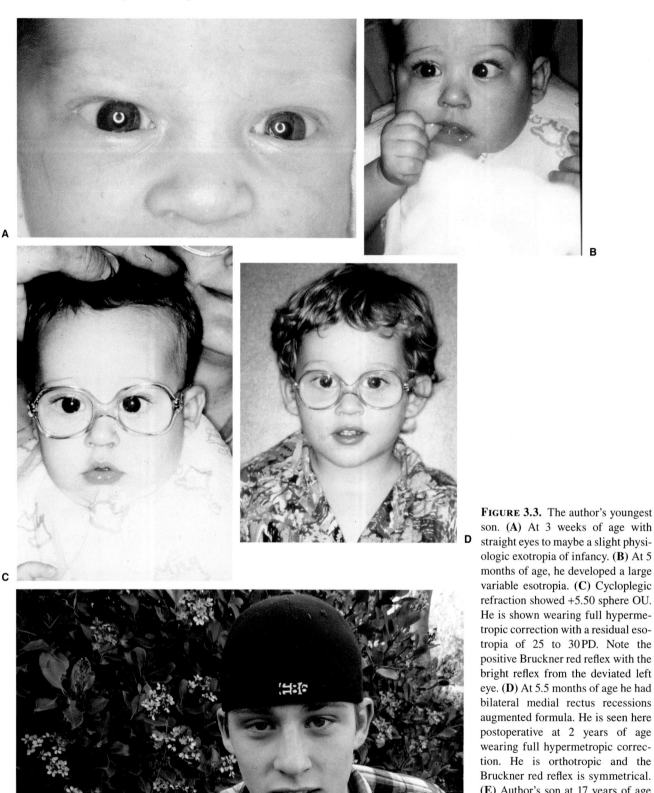

**FIGURE 3.3.** The author's youngest son. **(A)** At 3 weeks of age with straight eyes to maybe a slight physiologic exotropia of infancy. **(B)** At 5 months of age, he developed a large variable esotropia. **(C)** Cycloplegic refraction showed +5.50 sphere OU. He is shown wearing full hypermetropic correction with a residual esotropia of 25 to 30 PD. Note the positive Bruckner red reflex with the bright reflex from the deviated left eye. **(D)** At 5.5 months of age he had bilateral medial rectus recessions augmented formula. He is seen here postoperative at 2 years of age wearing full hypermetropic correction. He is orthotropic and the Bruckner red reflex is symmetrical. **(E)** Author's son at 17 years of age with straight eyes. He has high grade stereo acuity. He wore full hypermetropic correction until age 11 years when he grew out of the hypermetropic correction. Note this author treated his own son, including performing the strabismus surgery (less expensive that way).

spectacles at 3 months of age. If the eyes are aligned with spectacles, continue with the full hypermetropic correction. A residual esotropia after full hypermetropic correction requires a repeat cycloplegic refraction. Because of the young age, bifocal optical correction is not indicated in infantile accommodative esotropia. Evaluate for amblyopia and treat amblyopia after spectacles are prescribed. If a residual esotropia persists (>10 to 15 PD), after prescribing full hypermetropic correction, then surgery is indicated.

Do not reduce the plus unless an exophoria develops with correction. Reducing the plus will create a small esotropia and even a small esotropia disrupts binocular fusion. Some practitioners try to reduce the plus in order to "wean" the patient out of the spectacles. There is no data that indicates reducing the plus improves the hypermetropia or increases the chance of growing out of the spectacles. Importantly, the presence of even a small residual esotropia will interfere with binocular visual development and high grade stereo acuity.

A study by France and France from Wisconsin concluded that reducing the plus correction did not induce emmetropization. France stated: "It appears that the emmetropization that occurs in these patients (hypermetropic accommodative esotropia) is not dependent on the level of refractive correction."[6] This is the author's experience and, in fact, my son grew out of his hypermetropia at age 11 to 12, after wearing the full hypermetropic correction all his life.

**Indications for Surgery:** If a residual esotropia of >10 to 15 PD persists with full hypermetropic correction worn for 6 to 8 weeks, then surgery is indicated. Surgery is urgent as the longer the esotropia persists the worse the prognosis for establishing binocular fusion. Since infantile accommodative esotropia is acquired and the eyes are aligned during the early period of visual development, most patients have good binocular fusion potential.

**Surgical Procedure:** Distance measurements are difficult to obtain in infants so try to get a distance measurement, but base the surgery on the near deviation. Bilateral medial rectus muscle recessions are for a target angle between the deviation with and without hypermetropic correction.[7] The example below shows the augmented formula. See also Chapter 4 for other surgical formulas for accommodative esotropia.

---

*Example 3.2.  Clinical Example: Infantile Accommodative ET (see Figure 3.3)*

- 5-month old with a history of variable intermittent esotropia since 2 months of age (Figure 3.3). Now has a constant large angle esotropia.
- Strong fixation preference OD even with optical correction
- Ductions and versions normal
- Cycloplegic refraction
  OD +5.50 sphere
  OS +5.50 sphere

Nsc:     ET 55 PD        Ncc ET 25 PD    by prism cover test
Dsc:     ET 50 PD        Dcc ET 20 PD    by estimation
(D = distance, N = near, sc = without correction)

**Diagnosis:** Partially accommodative infantile esotropia (residual esotropia with optical correction, strabismic amblyopia left eye).

**Preoperative Treatment:** Prescribe full hypermetropic correction (+5.50 sphere OU). Patch right eye 4 to 6 hours a day and follow every week. Equal fixation preference was achieved with 2 weeks of patching, indicating resolution of amblyopia. After wearing full correction for 6 weeks and a repeat cycloplegic refraction, a residual esotropia of 25 PD persisted so strabismus surgery was planned.

**Surgery:** Bilateral medial rectus muscle recessions augmented surgery. Target angle is based on the near measurements as distance measurements are not reliable in infants. Average the near deviation with correction and the near deviation without correction: (55 + 25 / 2 = 40 PD target) or bilateral MR recessions 5.5 mm (see Appendix I on Surgical Numbers).

**Postoperative:** Postoperative day one variable small exotropia with correction. By the next day the exotropia disappeared, orthotropia for distance and near with full hypermetropic correction. Patient wore full hypermetropic correction (+5.50 sphere OU) and was orthotropic over 10 years. At 11 years of age patient grew out of hypermetropic correction over an 18 month period, and final cycloplegic refraction was +0.50 sphere. With 17 years of follow up patient has vision of 20/20 OU, high grade stereo acuity at least 100 seconds arc and orthotropia without correction (this is author's son).

**Surgical Goals:** The goal is to achieve orthotropia to establish high grade stereo acuity. We need to make every effort to align the eyes to within 8 to 10 PD for development and maintenance of binocular fusion. An esotropia larger than 8 to 10 PD will not allow binocular fusion (not even peripheral fusion), and should be considered for further treatment (see next section).

**Residual Esotropia:** The first step is to repeat the cycloplegic refraction. If there is more hypermetropia give the additional hypermetropic correction. If after prescribing full hypermetropic correction there is a residual ET >10 to 15 PD, then consider further surgery.

**Consecutive Exotropia:** An immediate small exodeviation (10 to 15 PD) is usually "good" as most will improve over several days to weeks because convergence amplitudes are strong. If the exotropia persists, try reducing the hypermetropic correction. Do not reduce the plus by more than +2.00 diopters as this leads to alignment instability. A consecutive exotropia lasting more than 2 to 3 months should be considered for a reoperation.

Consider the possibility of a medial rectus muscle dehiscence (stretched scar or slipped muscle) if the exotropia is associated with even a mild adduction deficit. In these cases explore the medial rectus muscles and advance it if there is an insertion dehiscence. Surgical management plan is same as for consecutive exotropia as discussed in congenital esotropia above.

## Other Issues on Infantile Esotropia

### Möbius syndrome

Möbius syndrome is facial diplegia and bilateral sixth nerve palsies (Figure 3.4). Limb and chest malformations have also been described. These children have a large angle esotropia with the eyes fixed in adduction. They have poor abduction and no abduction saccadic eye movements, thus the diagnosis of bilateral sixth nerve palsies is usually made. In reality it is likely that the limited abduction is not a true palsy as the medial rectus muscles are virtually always tight and abduction improves after surgery. It is more likely that the limited abduction is caused by tight fibrotic medial rectus muscles.

**Surgical Treatment**: One may think that a transposition procedure might be necessary because of the poor lateral rectus function, but these patients usually do very well with bilateral medial rectus recessions 6.0mm to 7.0mm.

### Esotropia, Latent Nystagmus, and Face Turn

Latent nystagmus is a nystagmus that is provoked when binocular vision is disrupted either by occluding one eye, or by the occurrence of a manifest strabismus. This nystagmus is characterized by the fast phase to the fixing eye and a null point in adduction. Esotropia, latent nystagmus, and face turn is seen in older patients with surgically corrected congenital esotropia.

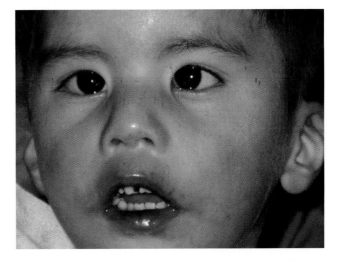

**FIGURE 3.4.** Patient with Möbius syndrome showing the typical lack of facial expression and esotropia.

They adopt a face turn to place the fixing eye in adduction to reduce the nystagmus and improve vision. The treatment is described in Chapter 6.

### Older Children and Adults with Infantile Esotropia

In general, adults or children older than 5 to 7 years, with uncorrected infantile esotropia, have a poor prognosis for binocular fusion. Even older patients, however, will occasionally show a surprise outcome of good binocular function and even stereo acuity.

### Treatment

- If there is poor fusion potential aim to undercorrect slightly, and leave an esotropia of 6 to 8 PD.
- If amblyopic (20/50 or worse), consider monocular surgery (MR recession and LR resection) on the amblyopic eye to avoid surgical risk to the "good" eye.

### Inferior Oblique Overaction

Inferior oblique overaction is usually bilateral and develops after 1 or 2 years of age. If significant overaction (+2 or more) is present on initial presentation of the esotropia, then perform inferior oblique muscle surgery concurrent with the horizontal surgery. Do not plan a separate staged second operation to weaken the inferior oblique muscles. An inferior oblique graded anteriorization is my procedure of choice as it reduces the V pattern, eliminates inferior oblique overaction, and reduces DVD. Do not modify the amount of horizontal surgery because of the inferior oblique weakening procedure. See Chapter 17 for further discussion on inferior oblique surgery.

### Dissociated Strabismus—Dissociated Vertical Deviation (DVD) and Dissociated Horizontal Deviation (DHD)

DVD is commonly associated with congenital esotropia, however over the last 10 years we have seen a drop in DVD severe enough to require surgery. This may be due to early surgery and better sensory outcomes. The indication for surgery for DVD or DHD is mostly based on the patient's cosmetic requirements. See Chapter 7 for details on the management of DVD and DHD.

## References

1. Pediatric Eye Disease Investigator Group. Spontaneous resolution of early-onset esotropia: experience of the Congenital Esotropia Observational Study. Am J Ophthalmol 2002;133:109–118.
2. Wright KW. Clinical optokinetic nystagmus asymmetry in treated esotropes. J Pediatr Ophthalmol Strabismus 1996;33:153–155.
3. Wright KW, Edelman PM, McVey JH, Terry AP, Lin M. High grade stereo acuity after early surgery for congenital esotropia. Arch Ophthalmol 1994;122:913–919.
4. Pediatric Eye Disease Investigator Group. The clinical spectrum of early-onset esotropia: experience of the Congenital Esotropia Observational Study. Am J Ophthalmol 2002;133:102–108.

5. Ciancia AO. Infantile esotropia with abduction nystagmus. Int Ophthalmol Clin 1989;29:24–29 (Review).
6. France TD, France LW, Orthoptics in Focus—Visions for the New Millennium. Transactions IX International Orthoptic Congress, Stockholm, Sweden,1999;223–226.
7. Wright KW, Bruce-Lyle L. Augmented surgery for esotropia associated with high hypermetropia. J Pediatr Ophthalmol Strabismus 1998;30:167–170.

# 4  Acquired Esotropia

Acquired esotropia requires an **_urgent consult_** for at least three important reasons:

1. Patients with acquired strabismus have fusion potential that diminishes in proportion to the duration of the esotropia. Early intervention can result in restoration of high grade binocular fusion.
2. Prompt dispensing of hypermetropic spectacle correction reduces the occurrence of amblyopia and increases the likelihood that spectacles alone will correct the esotropia, obviating the need for surgery.
3. Acquired esotropia can be a presenting sign of a neurological process such as myasthenia gravis, chronic progressive external ophthalmoplegia (CPEO), Arnold-Chiari malformation, or an intracranial tumor causing a sixth nerve paresis.

This chapter covers accommodative esotropia, non-accommodative acquired esotropia, cyclic esotropia, and sensory esotropia.

## Accommodative Esotropia

### Clinical Features

- Esotropia is usually acquired between 1 to 3 years of age but may occur in infancy (see Chapter 3)
- Variable moderate to large angle esotropia (20 to 50 PD)
- Initially intermittent then can progress to a constant esotropia
- Associated with hypermetropia usually +2.00 to +6.00 sphere

### Etiology

Hypermetropia associated with increased accommodation to achieve a clear image resulting in over convergence and esotropia.

### Clinical Evaluation

**Cycloplegic Refraction:** Use cyclopentolate 1% two doses, 5 minutes apart and refract 30 minutes after the last dose. Consider using atropine if the cycloplegia with cyclopentolate is inadequate.

**Amblyopia:** First prescribe the full hypermetropic correction. After wearing full correction for 4 weeks evaluate for fixation preference. Strong preference for one eye indicates amblyopia. Treat amblyopia by patching the dominant eye 4 to 6 hours a day until the patient holds fixation well with the nondominant eye.

**Measure Deviation:** Prism alternate cover test is most accurate and usually can be performed on these children. Use an accommodative target (i.e., a target with fine detail requiring full accommodation to see). The deviation should be measured for distance and near, with and without correction.

*Management*

The first step is to prescribe full hypermetropic correction and, second, to operate if there is a residual esotropia >10 to 15 PD and no fusion with full correction. Patients with accommodative esotropia usually have straight eyes during the early period of binocular visual development and become esotropic around 1 to 3 years of age. Since they had developed binocular fusion in infancy, they have the potential for binocular fusion and stereo acuity. Our goal is to align the eyes as soon as possible in order to re-establish binocular fusion and prevent amblyopia. Over time, cortical suppression associated with the esotropia will reduce binocular potential. In patients with strong fixation preference, cortical suppression will result in amblyopia of the nonpreferred eye. The late Dr. Marshall Parks considered acquired esotropia an urgent consult and would see these patients the same day they called for an appointment. The goal is to align the eyes and obtain binocular fusion, with patient wearing full hypermetropic correction. High-grade stereo acuity can be frequently achieved if early alignment is obtained.

**Optical Correction:** A refractive error significant enough to warrant spectacles is usually +2.00 sphere or more. Give the full hypermetropic correction as soon as the esodeviation is identified, even as early as 2 months of age. These patients accept their full correction. In most cases the family will notice a significant improvement in visual behavior with the spectacles. Do not reduce the plus unless an exophoria develops with correction. Remember, even a small esotropia disrupts binocular fusion. Some try to reduce the plus in order to wean the patient out of the spectacles. There is no data that indicates reducing the plus increases the chances to "grow out of spectacles". There is, however, data that shows the full plus correction will not interfere with the natural reduction of hypermetropia.[1] Reducing the plus usually produces a small esotropia compromising the development of binocular fusion.

Most children with accommodative esotropia will accept their spectacles if prescribed correctly. If a child objects to wearing hypermetropic spectacles, check the refraction. If the proper refraction was given and the child still refuses to wear the spectacles try giving atropine 0.5% (<2 years old) or 1% (older children) for 2 or 3 days to both eyes, to help children accept the full hypermetropic correction. Children must wear their spectacles full time for 4 to 6 weeks before deciding if the optical correction will correct the esotropia. Listed below are three responses to prescribing full hypermetropic spectacle correction for acquired accommodative esotropia.

*Responses to Hypermetropic Correction*

There are three common responses to prescribing hypermetropic spectacle correction for acquired accommodative esotropia.

1. Corrects the esotropia for both distance and near to within 8 PD
2. Corrects the esotropia for distance but there is a residual esotropia >10 PD for near
3. A residual esotropia >10 PD is present for both distance and near

**Esotropia Corrected Distance and Near:** If full hypermetropic spectacle correction results in a tropia <8 PD for distance and near, then single vision spectacles (without bifocals) are to be continued, and surgery is not indicated (Example 4.1). This is termed **accommodative esotropia**.

---

### Example 4.1.  Accommodative Esotropia

Cycloplegic refraction: +3.25 sphere OU
  Dsc ET 25 PD          Dcc E 2 PD
  Nsc ET 35 PD          Ncc E 4 PD
(D = distance, N = near, sc = without correction, cc = with correction)

Stereo acuity 100 seconds arc

**Treatment:** Single vision spectacles, no need for bifocals.

---

**Distance Corrected, but there is Residual Esotropia at Near (High AC/A Ratio):** If the full hypermetropic correction corrects the distance deviation resulting in fusion (i.e., ET <10 PD), but a residual esotropia persists at near that can not be fused (usually an ET >8 to 10 PD), then prescribe a **bifocal add**. These patients have a **high AC/A ratio accommodative esotropia** (Example 4.2). Prescribe the least amount of near add to obtain fusion and correct the near esotropia. Most patients will require +2.50 to +3.00 sphere add at the start. Example 4.2 below shows a perfect bifocal candidate: fusing in the distance with full hypermetropic correction and having an esotropia at near, but fuses at near with a +3.00 sphere bifocal add. Note that strabismus surgery is indicated if there is a significant esotropia in the distance that disrupts fusion, even if a bifocal add results in fusion at near. A flat top bifocal that splits the pupil is preferable until the child learns to use the bifocal well, then change to a progressive add if desired for cosmetic reasons.

---

### Example 4.2.  High AC/A Ratio Accommodative Esotropia (Bifocal Candidate)

Cycloplegic refraction +3.00 sphere OU, and full plus has been prescribed.
  Dcc E 2 PD (fusing)
  Ncc ET 35
  Ncc Bifocal +3.00 sphere add E 5 PD (fusing)
(D = distance, N = near, cc = with correction)

**Treatment:** Full hypermetropic correction with a bifocal add (+3.00 flat top add OU). Surgery is not required. Note: The AC/A ratio is 10 = [(35 − 5)/3]. This is a high AC/A ratio (normal AC/A ratio is 3 to 5).

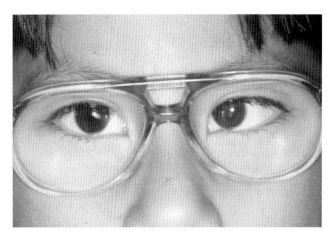

**FIGURE 4.1.** 7-year old with partially accommodative esotropia (residual esotropia >10 PD for distance and near with full hypermetropic correction). This patient requires strabismus surgery.

**Residual Esotropia Distance and Near (Partially Accommodative Esotropia):** If after prescribing the full hypermetropic correction, a distance esotropia persists, that cannot be fused (>10 PD), then surgery is indicated. This is termed partially accommodative esotropia. Remember, a bifocal add is not indicated if an esotropia persists in the distance that interferes with binocular fusion. These patients with a residual distance esotropia wearing full hypermetropic correction have partially accommodative esotropia and require strabismus surgery.

### Surgery for Partially Accommodative Esotropia

The surgical goal for partially accommodative esotropia is not to operate the patient out of spectacles, but to achieve alignment and fusion with full hypermetropic correction. Patients who have a cycloplegic refraction of +2.50 sphere or more will usually require their hypermetropic spectacles after surgery to maintain a stable result. Most authorities agree that bilateral medial rectus recessions (BMR) is the treatment of choice for partially accommodative esotropia. There are various strategies to determine the surgical target angle. The "standard" surgical strategy has been to operate for the residual esotropia measured in the distance while wearing full hypermetropic correction. Results with the standard approach have been disappointing, showing a high undercorrection rate of approximately 25% to 30%. Increasing the amount of surgery (e.g., augmented surgery formula or prism adaptation) improves results. The "augmented surgery formula" developed by the author has improved outcomes to over 90% alignment success rate with a minimum of 1 year follow-up in patients with a normal AC/A ratio accommodative esotropia.[2]

High AC/A ratio partially accommodative esotropia with a relatively small distance measurement and large near measurement is more difficult to manage as the distance to near discrepancy usually persists postoperatively. Some have advocated adding a faden to the medial rectus muscle recession to reduce the large near esotropia. In my experience the faden operation does not significantly reduce the AC/A ratio. This author prefers bilateral medial rectus recessions using a target angle based on the augmented formula with slight reduction of the numbers to prevent a consecutive exotropia for distance. Patients with high AC/A ratio partially accommodative esotropia should be informed that bifocal spectacles may be required after surgery.

Three methods for determining the target angle for partially accommodative ET are described below in Example 4.3.

---

## Example 4.3. Partially Accommodative Esotropia

3 year old
Cycloplegic refraction: +4.00 sphere OU
   Nsc ET 60 PD      Ncc ET 40 PD
   Dsc ET 50 PD      Dcc ET 30 PD
(D = distance, N = near, sc = without correction, cc = with correction)

---

### 1. Standard Surgery Formula
Target angle is the residual distance deviation with full hypermetropic correction.
*Example:* Dcc ET 30 PD
*Target Angle:* **30 PD**
*Surgery:* BMR recessions 4.5 mm

### 2. Augmented Surgery Formula
The target angle is an average between near deviation without correction and distance deviation with hypermetropic correction (average of the largest deviation and the smallest deviation).
*Example:* Average Nsc ET 60 PD and Dcc ET 30 PD
*Target Angle:* **45 PD**
*Surgery:* BMR recessions 5.75 mm

### 3. Prism Adaptation
The rationale for prism adaptation is that prism neutralization done over a long period of time will bring out the full latent deviation and reduce surgical undercorrection. It can also help to determine if the patient has fusion potential. Press-on prisms are prescribed to neutralize the distance deviation, and the patient wears them for 1 or 2 weeks, returning for re-measurement. If there is a residual esotropia with the press-on prisms, then the prisms are increased to neutralize the full esotropia, and the patient wears the new prisms for another 1 to 2 weeks. This process is repeated until the angle is stable. Surgery is based on the full prism adapted angle (Example 4.4).

> *Example 4.4  Prescribe 30 PD (distance deviation with correction) base out press-on prisms over full hypermetropic correction. Return visit in 1 week shows that with the press on prisms in place, the deviation now measures:*
>
>   Ncc ET 20 PD with prism (ET 50 total)
>   Dcc ET 15 PD with prism (ET 45 total)
> (D = distance, N = near, cc = with correction)
>
> Now prescribe 45 PD base out press-on prisms over full hyper-metropic correction and return in 1 week. At follow up visit, there is no change in the deviation, after placing the 45 PD base out prism (i.e., orthophoria with 45 PD base out prisms).
>
> *Target Angle:* **45 PD**
> *Surgery:* BMR recessions 5.75 mm

## Miotics for Accommodative Esotropia

Miotics are not a substitute for spectacles but in selected patients, miotic drops, such as phospholine iodide (i.e., Echothiophate Iodide), may be indicated to treat accommodative esotropia. Miotics reduce the AC/A ratio and esotropia associated with hypermetropia. Miotics can be tried if the patient has a high AC/A ratio, and has minimal hypermetropia. In most cases, however, bifocal spectacles are the treatment of choice. Another indication for the use of miotics is in children who cannot wear spectacles or contact lenses. This is most useful for short periods of time, such as during the summer months when children are swimming. When using miotics, it is preferable to start with a low dose of phospholine iodide, one drop of 0.03% every morning. If this dose is not sufficient to correct the esotropia, the dose may be increased to twice a day or use phospholine iodide 0.125%. Over the past 10 years the author (KWW) has used miotics once.

**Adverse Effects of Miotics:** Topical phospholine iodide prolongs the effect of succinylcholine and may prolong respiratory paralysis after surgery. Succinylcholine should be avoided if phospholine iodide has been used within 6 weeks prior to surgery. Systemic side effects of miotics may include brow ache, headache, nausea, and abdominal cramps. These complications are infrequent with low dose phospholine iodide. Ocular side effects of phospholine iodide include iris cysts along the pupillary margin in 20% to 50% of cases, which can occur anywhere from several weeks to several months after treatment. Iris cysts tend to regress after discontinuing phospholine iodide, however, this author has seen persistent iris cysts several years after stopping phospholine iodide therapy. Phenylephrine 2.5%, used in combination with phospholine iodide, may prevent iris cysts. Other rare and unusual complications include lens opacities, retinal detachment in adults, and angle closure glaucoma.

## *Postoperative Management of Partially Accommodative Esotropia—Surgical Goal*

Patients with accommodative esotropia have acquired strabismus and therefore, usually have good binocular fusion potential. The goal is deviation within 8 PD of orthotropia, to obtain binocular fusion with patient wearing full hypermetropic correction. High-grade stereopsis can be frequently achieved.

## *Residual Esotropia Distance and Near*

Repeat cycloplegic refraction and prescribe full hypermetropic correction. If an esotropia >10 to 15 PD persists in the distance and the child has fusion potential, then surgery is indicated.

- If primary surgery was bilateral MR recessions 5.0 mm or less, then re-recess MR (additional 2.0 mm recession OU corrects about 20 PD).
- If primary MR recession OU was >5.0 mm, then resect LR OU. Reduce the standard resection numbers by at least 1 mm to 2 mm, because you are resecting against a large MR recession and overcorrections are common in these cases.

## *Residual Esotropia Only at Near*

Patients with a preoperative high AC/A ratio will often have a residual esotropia at near after surgery and may require a bifocal add. If there is a residual esotropia at near (ET > 10 PD), but the eyes are aligned for distance, prescribe a bifocal add (+2.00 to +3.00 sphere) to establish comfortable fusion at near (see Example 4.2. High AC/A Ratio Accommodative Esotropia [Bifocal Candidate]).

## *Consecutive Exotropia*

For small angle consecutive exotropia, reduce hypermetropic correction to stimulate accommodative convergence. Reduction of more than +2.00 sphere usually results in angle instability and is not desirable. In the case of large angle consecutive exotropia consider reoperation. A large consecutive exotropia is unusual in these patients with partially accommodative esotropia, so consider the possibility of a slipped medial rectus muscle or stretched insertion scar, even if ductions are only slightly limited. In these cases advance the medial rectus muscles, as recessing the lateral rectus muscles will not provide stable alignment. (See Chapter 21 for Reoperation Techniques).

## Non-Accommodative Acquired Esotropia

Most often, a case of comitant acquired esotropia is simply a preexisting esophoria that has broken down into a tropia. Check for prisms in old glasses to identify that the deviation is long standing.

## *Clinical Features*

- Usually emmetropic, may be myopic
- Onset after 2 years—often late adulthood
- Full ductions
- Late onset ET of unknown etiology

*Differential Diagnosis*

- Breakdown of an esophoria (most common)
- Sixth nerve paresis (tumor, head trauma, or microvascular disease)
- Arnold Chiari malformation
- Hydrocephalus
- Aneurysm
- Myasthenia gravis
- Chronic progressive external ophthalmoplegia

**Divergence Paresis Pattern:** An esotropia with a distance deviation greater than near is a divergence paresis pattern. This is a common pattern of acquired esotropia in adults over 40 years old. A divergence paresis pattern may indicate a sixth nerve paresis and possible neurological disease. Consider a neurological evaluation and neuro-imaging especially if the deviation is incomitant or abduction is limited. The vast majority of patients with divergence paresis esotropia and full ductions will have a negative neurological work-up. Adults with a well documented long standing esotropia and horizontal comitance usually do not require an extensive neurological work-up.

**Treatment:** In patients with a comitant acquired esotropia, perform bilateral medial rectus recessions. Surgery for acquired esotropia often results in an undercorrection, so increase the amount of recession. Try using prism adaptation to determine the full target angle, especially if there is a disparity between the distance and near deviation. Operate for the full prism adapted angle (see prism adaptation). If an adjustable suture is used, adjust to a slight overcorrection of exophoria 5 to 10 PD.

## Cyclic Esotropia

*Clinical Features*

- Acquired ET in childhood
- Cyclic pattern: some days esotropic; other days orthotropic
- Progresses to constant tropia phase

Cyclic esotropia is a rare type of acquired esotropia. It can occur at virtually any age, but most frequently occurs between 2 to 6 years of age. These patients cycle between straight eyes and esotropia (see Figure 4.2). Various patterns are possible and the intervals between being esotropic and orthotropic are not always exactly the same. When the eyes are aligned, the patient has good binocular vision and stereo acuity, but usually suppresses when tropic. Cyclic esotropia is usually progressive, and most will become a constant tropia over several months to even years. Some cases of cyclic esotropia are associated with hypermetropia and, in these cases the full cycloplegic correction should be given.

*Treatment*

- Prescribe full hypermetropic correction if +1.50 sphere or more.
- Perform surgery if spectacles do not correct the esotropia. Operate for the full deviation measured on the esotropic day.

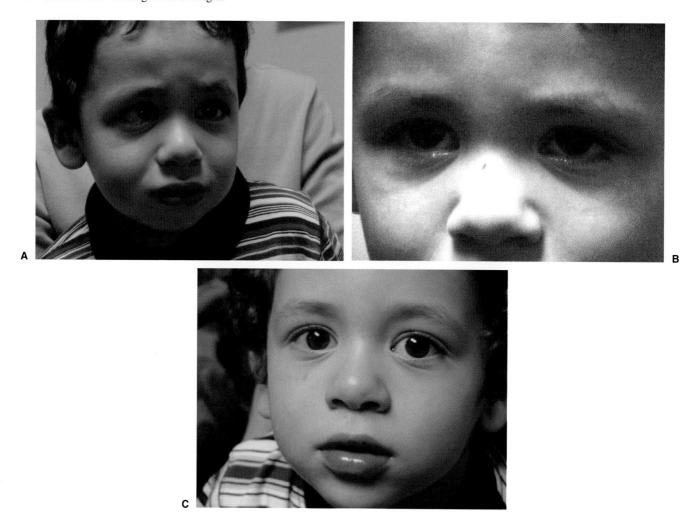

**FIGURE 4.2.** **(A)** A preoperative photograph of a patient with cyclic esotropia. The patient had a large angle esotropia this day: "A crossed eyed day!" **(B)** A preoperative photograph of a patient with cyclic esotropia. The patient was orthotropic this day: "A straight eyed day!" Despite straight eyes on the day of surgery large bilateral medial rectus muscle recession was done. **(C)** Postoperative photograph showing straight eyes after large bilateral medical rectus recessions. The patient was operated for the full esodeviation seen on a crossed eyed day, despite the fact the patient was orthophoric to alternate cover test the day of surgery. The family was very pleased with the surgical result: "orthotropia."

## Sensory Esotropia

Sensory esotropia is associated with a monocular poor vision of usually 20/100 or worse.

### Clinical Evaluation

Patients with poor vision do not fixate well, therefore, prism cover testing will not be accurate. If ductions are full you can estimate the deviation by placing the appropriate base out prism over the "good" eye to move the amblyopic eye out to a cosmetically acceptable primary position (Hering's law). Estimate the deviation for distance by placing a base out prism over the good eye to move the deviated eye to primary position. If ductions are limited, use the Krimsky test for near with the prism over the deviated eye.

*Treatment*

Perform monocular surgery on the poor vision eye, specifically, a medial rectus recession and lateral rectus tightening procedure (plication or resection). Use the standard surgical numbers from the chart (see Appendix I).

# References

1. France TD, France LW. Orthoptics in focus-visions for the new millennium. Transactions IX International Orthoptic Congress. Stockholm; 1999:223–226.
2. Wright KW, Bruce-Lyle L. Augmented surgery for esotropia associated with high hypermetropia. J Pediatr Ophthalmol Strabismus 1998;30:167–170.

# 5 Exotropia

## Intermittent Exotropia—X(T)

Intermittent exotropia is a large exophoria that intermittently breaks down to an exotropia. Occluding one eye breaks fusion and will manifest the exotropia (Figure 5.1). When fusing, the eyes are straight and stereo acuity is excellent, usually 40 seconds of arc. When tropic, there is large hemi-retinal suppression of the deviated eye. It is common for patients to show a preference for one eye, however, resist the temptation to label the deviation as a right or left exotropia. You can easily change the deviated eye by covering the dominant eye. Patients with late onset exotropia during late childhood or adulthood may experience diplopia when tropic. The exotropia is typically manifest when the patient is fatigued, daydreaming or ill. Approximately 80% of intermittent exotropia patients will show progressive loss of fusion control and an increase in the exotropia over several months to years. Adult patients can have extremely large deviations (Figure 5.2). The patient in Figure 5.2 has alternating intermittent exotropia. Despite the large angle exotropia she was able to fuse intermittently.

### Clinical Features

- Most common form of exotropia
- Usually presents after 1 year of age
- Large exophoria (usually 25 to 40 PD) that spontaneously becomes manifest
- High grade stereo acuity when fusing (40 seconds arc); suppression when tropic
- Squints one eye to bright light
- High hypermetropia with exotropia (rare subtype of intermittent exotropia)

### Etiology

The cause of the underlying exotropia is unknown, but the control of the deviation and the high grade stereo acuity can be explained on the basis of strong fusional convergence. Fusional convergence is naturally strong (25 to 30 PD), so exodeviations are better controlled than esodeviations as divergence amplitudes are small (6 to 8 PD).

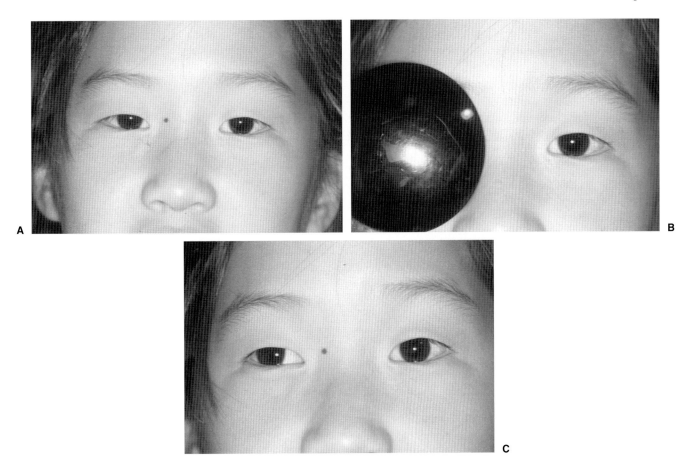

**FIGURE 5.1.** Child with an intermittent exotropia. **(A)** Shows patient with intermittent exotropia fusing with straight eyes. **(B)** Cover over right eye to dissociate the eyes and break fusion. **(C)** Fusion is broken and patient manifests the latent exotropia.

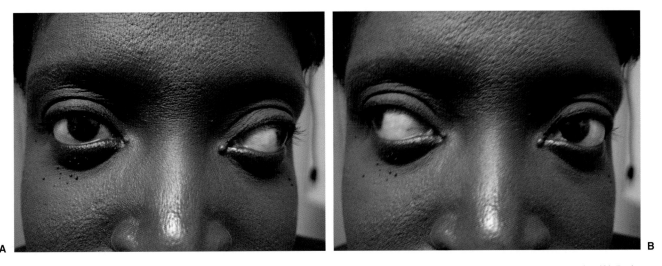

**FIGURE 5.2.** Adult patient with childhood intermittent exotropia that increased over time to a large angle constant exotropia. **(A)** Patient is fixing with the right eye, left eye deviated. **(B)** Patient is fixing with the left eye, right eye deviated.

*Clinical Evaluation*

**Ductions:** Adduction should be full.

**Versions:** Check for oblique dysfunction and "A" or "V" patterns.

**Amblyopia:** Amblyopia can occur but is rare, usually associated with anisometropia. If decreased vision is present, think about an organic cause (e.g., optic nerve disease).

**Measure the Deviation:** Use prolonged prism alternate cover testing for far distance fixation (at least 20 feet) and near fixating on an accommodative target, to measure the deviation. Prolonged cover testing helps to break down tonic fusion and reveal the full deviation. Consider the patch test for patients with a divergence excess pattern (see divergence excess below).

**Cycloplegic Refraction:** A cycloplegic refraction is important as high hypermetropia with hypoaccommodation can cause an intermittent exodeviation. The treatment is to prescribe the full hypermetropic correction.

*Nonsurgical Treatment*

In general, nonsurgical treatment does not work very well for intermittent exotropia. Indications for nonsurgical treatment include convergence insufficiency, small angle exophoria, interim treatment prior to surgery and high hypermetropia with exotropia.

*Nonsurgical Therapies*

- Part time monocular occlusion of the dominant eye, 3 to 4 hours a day. This is a form of anti-suppression therapy that works by stimulating the nonpreferred eye. In patients with equal ocular preference, alternate eye patching is indicated.
- Over minus: Prescribe −1.50 to −2.50 sphere more than required by cyclopegic refraction. This will increase accommodative convergence and may help to control the intermittent exotropia. It is usually only effective for small deviations in myopic patients.
- Orthoptics: Convergence exercises (pencil push-ups or base out prisms) are the treatment of choice for convergence insufficiency. Orthoptics are usually not helpful for correcting the distance exodeviation.

## High Hypermetropia with Exotropia

Patients with hypermetropia (>+4.00 sphere OU) may present with a small exotropia. These patients have some degree of bilateral amblyopia and are hypoaccommodators. Their small exotropia is secondary to poor accommodation and deficient convergence. Treatment is to prescribe the full hypermetropic correction. By prescribing the full plus, vision and accommodation improve, thus improving convergence and control of the exotropia. Surgery is indicated if there is a residual exotropia after prescribing full hypermetropic correction. Do not be afraid to prescribe the full plus!

*Preoperative Evaluation*

### Indications for Surgery

- Increasing tropia phase with diminished fusion control.
- Poor fusion recovery on cover/uncover testing.
- Exotropia that is manifested more than 50% of waking hours.
- The size of the deviation is of less importance but, in most cases, the exotropia should be >15 PD.

### Children Under 4 Years of Age

Children under 4 years of age are at risk of developing postoperative amblyopia from a consecutive esotropia. It is probably best to postpone surgery until 4 years of age unless the patient demonstrates progressive loss of fusion control. A consecutive esotropia in these young children must be followed closely to check for development of postoperative amblyopia.

*Surgical Treatment*

The procedure of choice for all types of intermittent exotropia (see classification later in this chapter) is bilateral lateral rectus recessions. Symmetrical surgery is preferred over a monocular recession-resection procedure because the deviation is comitant and bilateral surgery gives a comitant result. A recession-resection procedure, on the other hand, causes horizontal incomitance, inducing an esotropia and diplopia on gaze to the side of the recession–resection. The incomitance may partially dissipate over time, but adults often complain of persistent diplopia on side gaze.

Small hyperphorias (<5 PD) are commonly associated with intermittent exotropia. These small hyperphorias can be ignored if they are not associated with oblique dysfunction, as they disappear after correction of the exotropia with bilateral lateral rectus recessions.

*Classification of Intermittent Exotropia*

Intermittent exotropia can be classified into three types based on the difference between the distance and near deviation: (1) basic, (2) divergence excess (pseudo and true), and (3) convergence insufficiency. This classification is clinically important as it helps determine the treatment.

1. **Basic X(T):** The distance and near deviations are similar, within 10 PD. The target angle is the distance deviation.

---

### Example 5.1. Basic X(T)

Distance        X(T) 35 PD
Near            X(T) 30 PD
Target angle: X(T) 35 PD
Surgery: Bilateral lateral rectus recessions 7.5 mm

**2. Divergence Excess Pattern:** The exotropia is larger for distance fixation than near fixation (>10 PD).

More than half of intermittent exotropia patients will have a divergence excess pattern, with the distance deviation being 10 PD larger that the near deviation. There are two types of divergence excess pattern intermittent exotropia: **true divergence excess** and **pseudo-divergence excess**. True divergence excess is when the divergence excess persists even after prolonged binocular dissociation by monocular patching (i.e., patch test). Pseudo-divergence excess is when the near deviation increases after the patch test so the distance and near deviations are similar. The vast majority of divergence excess pattern cases are pseudo-divergence excess. Patients with divergence excess intermittent exotropia should have a patch test to differentiate true from pseudo-divergence excess. Distinguishing true divergence excess from pseudo-divergence excess helps determine the target angle.

**Patch Test:** The patch test consists of patching one eye for 30 to 60 minutes, then measuring the deviation at distance and near without allowing the patient to reestablish fusion. Prolonged occlusion of one eye suspends tonic fusional convergence (same as tenacious proximal convergence) and reveals the full exophoria. Below are examples of true and pseudo-divergence excess intermittent exotropia.

**Pseudo-Divergence Excess:** Pseudo-divergence means the near exodeviation will increase to within 10 PD of distance exodeviation after prolonged monocular occlusion (patch test). Pseudo-divergence excess is caused by increased near tonic fusional convergence. Surgery is based on the distance deviation after the patch test as shown in the example below.

---

### Example 5.2.  Pseudo-Divergence Excess

| Distance | X(T) 35 PD |
| Near | X(T) 10 PD |

**After Patch Test**

| Distance | X(T) 35 PD RH 3 PD |
| Near | X(T) 30 PD |

Target angle: X(T) 30 to 35 PD

Surgery: Bilateral lateral rectus recessions between 7.0 and 7.5 mm

*Note*: Small hypertropias may be disclosed after prolonged dissociation. Disregard small hypertropias associated with intermittent exotropia as they will disappear after the exotropia is surgically corrected.

---

**True Divergence Excess:** This is an uncommon pattern of intermittent exotropia where the distance deviation is at least 10 PD larger than the near deviation even after the patch test. True divergence excess patients have a high AC/A ratio, and the near deviation increases with +3.00 sphere near add. A better term for these patients would be **high AC/A ratio intermittent exotropia**. The high AC/A ratio usually persists postoperatively, and can lead to a consecutive esotropia at near that may require a near add. The target angle in patients with true divergence excess should be an average of the distance and near deviation after the patch test.

---

### Example 5.3. True Divergence Excess

| | |
|---|---|
| Distance | X(T) 35 PD |
| Near | X(T) 10 PD |

**After patch test**

| | |
|---|---|
| Distance | X(T) 35 PD |
| Near | X(T) 15 PD |

Target angle: Between distance deviation (XT 35 PD) and near deviation after patch test (XT 15 PD); (35 + 15)/2 = target angle X(T) 25 PD

Surgery: Bilateral lateral rectus recessions 6.0 mm

---

**Important Note:** It is prudent to warn patients with true divergence excess having a high AC/A ratio that bifocal glasses may be needed postoperatively. Operating between the distance and near deviation produces a compromise and may result in a residual exotropia in the distance and a consecutive esotropia at near. These are very difficult cases and often require reoperation or settling for an imperfect result. Using prism adaptation by prescribing base in press-on prisms for the distance deviation may help predict if there will be a persistent ET at near and may also help determine the target angle.

### 3. Convergence Insufficiency

Convergence insufficiency is when the near deviation is at least 10 PD larger than the distance deviation. If there is no significant distance deviation, with an exodeviation for near, then this is a pure convergence insufficiency. These patients are best treated with orthoptic therapy (convergence exercises such as pencil push-ups) not surgery. Note that some have advocated medial rectus resections to enhance convergence in these patients. Rectus muscle resections, however, do not increase muscle function as resections create a leash. Thus, medial rectus muscle resections do not improve convergence; they limit divergence and usually create a distance esotropia and postoperative diplopia for distance fixation. In older patients unable to improve with convergence exercises, base out prisms in the reading spectacles can sometimes improve asthenopic symptoms. Prescribe the minimum amount of prism that allows for comfortable binocular fusion.

For patients with a significant intermittent exotropia (>15 PD) in the distance, associated with a larger near exotropia, surgery plus convergence exercises are indicated. It is a good idea to give convergence exercises prior to surgery and explain to the patient that postoperative exercises will probably be necessary.

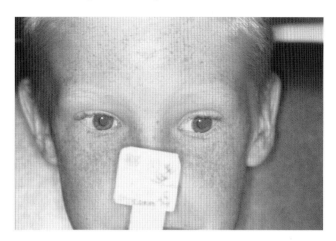

**FIGURE 5.3.** shows a patient with convergence insufficiency and remote near point of convergence.

---

## Example 5.4. Pure Convergence Insufficiency

Distance          Orthotropia
Near              X(T) 25 PD
Remote near point of convergence.

**Treatment:** Orthoptic convergence exercises: pencil push-ups, 20 repetitions, 3 times a day.

---

## Example 5.5. Intermittent Exotropia with Convergence Insufficiency

Distance          X(T) 20 PD
Near              X(T) 30 PD

Target angle between X(T) 20 to 30 PD (i.e., X(T) 25 PD) and post-operative convergence exercises.

**Treatment:** Preoperative convergence exercises, then bilateral lateral rectus recessions 6.0 mm and postoperative convergence exercises.

---

*Intermittent Exotropia: Oblique Overaction and A and V Patterns*

### V-Pattern

- If inferior oblique overaction is +2 or more with a V-pattern, then perform inferior oblique weakening procedures (usually bilateral) along with the lateral rectus recessions. Do not change the amount of horizontal surgery because of inferior oblique muscle surgery (see Chapter 17 for more information on inferior oblique weakening procedures).

- If there is no significant inferior oblique overaction, transpose the lateral recti superiorly one-half tendon width.

### A-Pattern

- For a small to moderate A-pattern with or without significant superior oblique overaction, perform bilateral lateral rectus recessions and transpose the lateral recti inferiorly one-half tendon width. Avoid superior oblique weakening procedures especially uncontrolled procedures such as tenotomy.
- For a large A-pattern with severe bilateral superior oblique overaction (+3 to +4) transpose the lateral recti inferiorly one-half tendon width and perform a controlled bilateral superior oblique weakening procedure such as the Wright silicone tendon expander (approximately 4 mm to 5 mm) or a split tendon elongation.

*Note:* Intermittent exotropia associated with superior oblique overaction and A-pattern is a difficult situation because superior oblique weakening procedures can lead to superior oblique palsy and diplopia in these patients with bifoveal fusion. Avoid uncontrolled superior oblique weakening procedures such as tenotomy, in favor of either a horizontal muscle vertical transposition (move the lateral recti inferiorly, see Chapter 15), or perform a controlled superior oblique tendon lengthening procedure such as the Wright silicone tendon expander (Chapter 19).

### X-Pattern

Another pattern often associated with intermittent exotropia is an X-pattern, having an increasing exodeviation in up gaze and down gaze relative to primary position. X-pattern may be associated with oblique dysfunction, however, in most cases there is no true oblique muscle overaction. The X-pattern usually disappears after bilateral lateral rectus recessions without doing oblique muscle surgery.

#### Postoperative Management

The immediate postoperative goal is to achieve a small consecutive esodeviation approximately 8 to 15 PD. Children under 4 years of age are prone to develop amblyopia, so part time alternate eye occlusion therapy may be used to prevent amblyopia until the esotropia resolves. In older patients, the initial consecutive esotropia usually causes diplopia. It is important to inform patients that transient diplopia frequently occurs after surgery. Hardesty has suggested prescribing prism glasses to neutralize the consecutive esodeviation early on in the postoperative course. He recommended prescribing prisms that leave a small esophoria to stimulate divergence.[1]

**Consecutive Esotropia:** If a consecutive esotropia persists for more than one week without fusion at distance or near, consider prescribing base out prisms (usually press-on) to stimulate fusion. Prescribe the least amount of base out prism that allows fusion, and leave an esophoria to stimulate divergence. Persistent esodeviations at near are frequent in patients with true divergence excess and a high AC/A ratio. These patients may require long-term bifocals. A persistent esodeviation present at six weeks after surgery, not controlled by conservative measures, should be considered for reoperation. In most cases, bilateral medial rectus recessions are indicated for small angle consecutive esotropia. Consider a slipped or stretched lateral rectus muscle if there is a large angle consecutive esotropia especially if abduction is limited (see Chapter 21).

**Residual Exotropia:** A residual exotropia is a common occurrence and usually occurs late, several months to years after the initial surgery. Indications for operating on a residual intermittent exotropia are similar to the initial surgery. For a residual exotropia of less than 6.0 mm, that occurs after lateral rectus recessions consider re-recessing both lateral rectus muscles (3.0 mm corrects about 20 PD). If the primary recessions were greater than 6.0 mm, consider bilateral medial rectus resections or plications. Be conservative about the amount of medial rectus tightening, as you are tightening against previously recessed lateral rectus muscles and this can cause a consecutive esotropia. Take 1.0 mm to 1.5 mm off the standard charts.

## Sensory XT

Vision loss after 2 years of age will often cause an exotropia and this is termed sensory exotropia. Surgery is for cosmetic indications. Monocular surgery on the poor vision eye is suggested to protect the "good eye": recess the lateral rectus muscle and tighten the medial rectus by a resection or plication.

## Congenital XT

Congenital exotropia is rare and occurs in the first few weeks of life. Like congenital esotropia, congenital exotropia patients have poor fusion potential. There is often an associated neurological or systemic disorder such as arthogryposis, albinism, or craniosynostosis (Figure 5.4).

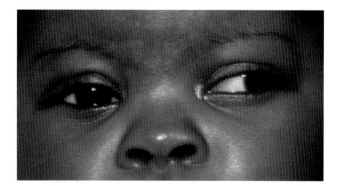

**FIGURE 5.4.** An infant with congenital exotropia associated with craniosynostosis.

*Clinical Features*

- Rare
- Onset by 6 months of age, usually present at birth
- Constant exotropia
- Large angle >40 PD

*Etiology*

Unknown

*Treatment*

- Correct amblyopia if present.
- Surgery for XT after 6 months of age, do bilateral lateral rectus recessions.

# Reference

1. Hardesty HH, Boynton JR, Keenan JP. Treatment of intermittent exotropia. Arch Ophthalmol 1978;96:268–274.

# 6 Torticollis, Nystagmus, and Incomitant Strabismus

## Torticollis: Compensatory Head Posturing

Torticollis comes from the Latin word *torti*, meaning twisted, and *collis*, meaning neck. Simplistically, we can consider two types of torticollis: musculoskeletal and ocular. Musculoskeletal torticollis is caused by tight neck muscles, usually the sternocleidomastoid, or a skeletal deformity. With musculoskeletal torticollis, the neck will resist passive flexion with the eyes open or closed, and these patients maintain their head posturing even during sleep. In contrast, ocular torticollis is a compensatory mechanism to achieve optimal vision in patients with nystagmus or incomitant strabismus. A face turn or head tilt is adopted to place the eyes in a position that either reduces nystagmus or improves eye alignment. Ocular torticollis may be horizontal (face turn), vertical (chin up or down), torsional (head tilt right or left), or a combination of the three. The best way to identify the presence of a face turn or chin posturing is by looking at the position of the eyes. A gaze preference indicates a face turn. For example, does the patient in Figure 6.1 have a face turn?

**Answer:** Yes! This patient has a compensatory face turn to the left, to keep the eyes in right gaze. This right gaze preference could be the result of nystagmus with a null point in right gaze or an incomitant strabismus with orthotropia in right gaze. The key to assessing a compensatory face turn is to observe the position of the eyes. If the eyes remain in an eccentric gaze then the face is turned.

### Strabismic Torticollis

**Incomitant strabismus** means the eyes are not moving in synchrony and this can be caused by ocular restriction, extraocular muscle paresis, extraocular muscle overaction, or A and V patterns. Patients with incomitant strabismus may adopt a face turn, a chin posture, or a head tilt to place the eyes in a position of alignment and achieve binocular fusion. For example, patients with a right congenital fourth nerve paresis will tilt their head to the left to reduce the hypertropia and maintain binocular fusion. Incomitant horizontal strabismus can cause a face turn. A tight medial rectus (MR) muscle in the right eye will produce an esotropia in right gaze and provoke a face turn to the right to keep the eyes aligned in left gaze.

The strategy for correcting a face turn caused by an incomitant strabismus is to correct the strabismus in primary position, and to increase the field of binocular fusion by improving the incomitance. If the ductions are relatively full, surgery can be done on either or both eyes to correct the

52

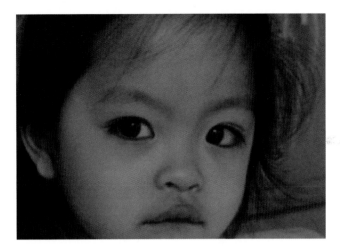

FIGURE 6.1. Patient with a compensatory face turn.

incomitance. If there is only minimal limitation it is often best to match the limitation by operating on the "good eye." In cases with significant limitation of movement of one eye (restriction or muscle palsy), correct the face turn by moving the eye with limited ductions into primary position. It does not help to operate on the normal eye if the eye with limited ductions can not move easily to the primary position. Below are examples for the treatment of incomitant strabismus causing a compensatory head posture.

### Example 1. Strabismus, Face Turn with Full Ductions

The patient in Figure 6.2 has a right partial sixth nerve paresis, good lateral rectus (LR) function, and full ductions.

Preoperative deviation

| Right gaze | Primary position | Left gaze |
|---|---|---|
| ET 25 PD | ET 15 PD | E 2 PD fusing |

The esotropia increases in right gaze so the patient maintains a compensatory face turn to the right to keep the eyes aligned in left gaze. The following are two treatment options to correct this strabismus and face turn.

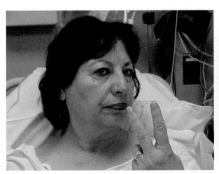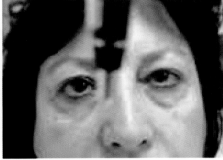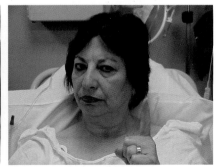

FIGURE 6.2. Patient with a right partial sixth nerve paresis and good lateral rectus function. Left figure shows patient with an esotropia and diplopia in right gaze. Right figure shows the patient with a compensatory face turn to the right to achieve single vision.

### *Option 1. Operate on the Paretic Eye*

Surgery: Right MR recession and right LR resection

|  | Right gaze | Primary position | Left gaze |
|---|---|---|---|
| Result: | ET 10 PD | Orthotropia | XT 12 PD |

### *Option 2. Asymmetric Bilateral Surgery: Operate on the Good Eye*

Surgery: Right MR recession 3 mm and left MR recession 6 mm

|  | Right gaze | Primary position | Left gaze |
|---|---|---|---|
| Result: | E2 PD | Orthotropia | X2 PD |

In this case the right lateral rectus is underacting so the left MR is overacting (Hering's law), producing an esotropia greater in right gaze. In option one, recessing the medial rectus and resecting the lateral rectus of the right eye does not improve abduction but limits adduction (see Chapter 2). Limiting adduction in the right eye induces an exotropia in left gaze and undercorrects the esotropia in right gaze. Option two is a better choice to provide the largest area of binocular single vision. A large left medial rectus recession reduces adduction slightly and that matches the slight abduction deficit of the right eye. This strategy of matching the function of yoke muscles (Hering's law) can be used in a wide range of incomitant strabismus cases, as long as the ductions are full or only slightly limited. Another aspect is that the left medial rectus recession has most of its effect in right gaze where the esodeviation is greatest. (See Chapter 2 for surgical correction of incomitant strabismus).

### *Example 2. Strabismus, Face Turn with Limited Ductions*

If the face turn is due to limited ductions of one eye and the eye is fixed in an eccentric position of gaze, simply move the eye with limited ductions into primary position. In the case in Figure 6.3 the left eye is in a position of rest in abduction because the left medial rectus muscle has slipped from previous strabismus surgery (elsewhere of course). The treatment is to advance the left MR muscle and recess the tight LR muscle to move the left eye into primary position. Once adduction of the left eye has improved, then consider surgery on the right eye (LR recession) to correct the antici-

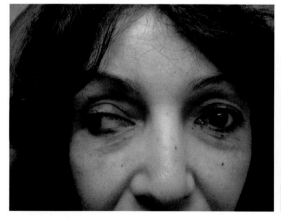 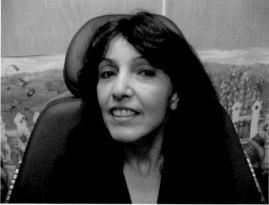

FIGURE 6.3. (Left) A patient with limited adduction in left eye, and left eye has difficulty coming to the midline because of a slipped medial rectus muscle. (Right) The same patient with a compensatory face turn to the right to keep the eyes aligned in left gaze where the left eye is in its position of rest.

pated residual exotropia in right gaze. Surgery on the good eye to reduce the overshoot (Hering's law), can be done primarily with the first surgery or as a secondary procedure.

### Example 3. Chin Up Head Posture with Limited Ductions

Patient has a left orbital **floor fracture** and had previous repair done but still has a tight left inferior rectus muscle. Patient has binocular single vision in down gaze and diplopia increasing in up gaze.

Preoperative deviation
Ductions:     Right eye—Full         Left eye—Limitation of elevation −1
              Up gaze                RHT 18 PD
              Primary position       RHT 9 PD
              Down gaze              Orthotropia

Surgery:      Bilateral Inferior rectus recessions (asymmetric)
              RE 3.5 mm, LE 4.5 mm
              Right Superior rectus recession 4.0 mm

Postoperative deviation
Ductions: Full in both eyes.
              Up gaze                RHT 4 PD
              Primary position       Orthotropia
              Down gaze              Orthotropia

The challenge is to improve the diplopia in primary position and up gaze without causing diplopia in down gaze. A recession of the tight left inferior rectus muscle will improve the deviation in up gaze, but will induce a left hypertropia in down gaze. Remember a recession has its greatest effect towards the recessed muscle. A better choice is bilateral asymmetric inferior rectus recessions with a contralateral (right) superior rectus recession. The bilateral inferior rectus recessions will not induce a vertical deviation in down gaze but will improve elevation. The contralateral superior rectus recession is most effective in up gaze, so it corrects the hypertropia in primary position that increases in up gaze.

## Torticollis and Nystagmus

Patients with nystagmus usually have a position of gaze where the nystagmus is least. This is the null point or null zone. If the null point is eccentric to primary position, the patient will adopt a compensatory face posture to place the eyes at the null point, in order to dampen the nystagmus and improve vision. The compensatory head posturing may be a face turn right or left, chin elevation or depression, head tilt, or a combination. A patient with a null point in down gaze will adopt a chin elevation to keep the eyes in down gaze. A null point in right gaze causes a face turn to the left, eyes to the right. The treatment for nystagmus related head posturing is based on using eye muscle surgery to move the eyes into primary position. Treat example below of right null point—face turn left by moving both eyes to the left into primary position (left eye: recess MR and resect LR; right eye: resect MR and recess LR) (Figure 6.4). This procedure is termed the Parks–Kestenbaum procedure. Table 6.1 provides surgical numbers for the Kestenbaum procedure, for various degrees of left face turn, eyes right.

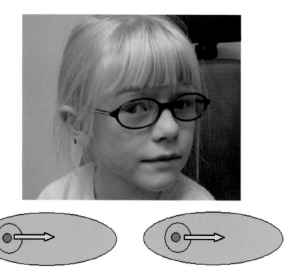

**FIGURE 6.4.** Eyes in right gaze at null point: Face turn left. Correct the face turn by surgically moving the eyes left into primary position.

**TABLE 6.1.** Parks–Kestenbaum Procedure

| | Null point right (eyes shifted right): Left face turn | | | |
|---|---|---|---|---|
| | Right eye | | Left eye | |
| Left face turn (degrees) | Recess lateral rectus (mm) | Resect medial rectus (mm) | Recess medial rectus (mm) | Resect lateral rectus (mm) |
| <20 | 7 | 6 | 5 | 8 |
| 30 | 9 | 8 | 6.5 | 10 |
| 45 | 10 | 8.5 | 7 | 11 |
| >50 | 11 | 9.5 | 8 | 12.5 |

The surgical numbers are large as the goal is to create a limitation of eye movements to shift the null point. An initial overcorrection is desirable, as the face turn tends to recur.

*Correcting Strabismus Associated with Nystagmus and Face Turn*

Some patients will have strabismus associated with congenital nystagmus and face turn. These patients pose a special challenge. First identify the fixing eye and its null point as this determines the face turn. The strategy is to: 1) move the fixing eye to primary position and 2) correct any residual or induced strabismus by moving the nonfixing eye (Figure 6.5).

**Surgical Strategy**

1. Move the null point of the fixing eye (left eye) to primary position for a face turn of 30 degrees

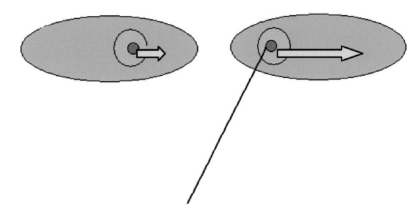

FIGURE 6.5. Patient with esotropia and nystagmus fixing with the left eye at the null point in adduction. There is a left face turn of 30 degrees and an esotropia of 40 PD. Long Arrow shows moving the fixing eye (left) a lot for the face turn, and the short arrow indicates moving the non-fixing eye (right) a little to correct the consecutive exotropia.

*Left eye:* Recess the MR 6.5 mm and resect the LR 10 mm (i.e., Parks numbers for Kestenbaum).

2. Move the non-fixing eye (right eye) to correct the residual or induced strabismus as a result of moving the fixing eye. Since the esotropia measures 40 PD, and the large MR recession 6.5 mm + LR resection 10.0 mm left eye corrects about 70 PD of esotropia (see Appendix I on Surgical Numbers—monocular), an exotropia of about 30 PD would be induced. We need to correct for this anticipated exotropic shift of 30 PD by simultaneously moving the right eye in for 30 PD.

*Right eye:* Recess LR 6.5 mm and resect MR 5.0 mm.

### Summary

*Left eye:* Recess MR 6.5 mm, and resect LR 10 mm.
*Right eye:* Recess LR 6.5 mm and resect MR 5.0 mm.

### Manifest Latent Nystagmus with Esotropia and Face Turn

Latent nystagmus is a nystagmus that is provoked when binocular vision is disrupted either by occluding one eye, or by the occurrence of a manifest strabismus. This nystagmus is characterized by the fast phase to the fixing eye and a null point in adduction. A latent nystagmus that becomes manifest is termed manifest latent nystagmus (MLN). When a patient develops MLN they adopt a face turn to place the fixing eye in adduction to reduce the nystagmus and improve vision. Latent nystagmus is associated with disorders that disrupt binocular visual development including congenital esotropia, and monocular congenital cataracts. Clinically we see MLN with esotropia and face turn in older patients with surgically corrected congenital esotropia. These patients have peripheral fusion and an esophoria. At times their esophoria will break down into a tropia, and the latent nystagmus will become manifest. To reduce the manifest latent nystagmus and improve vision, the patient adopts a face turn to place the fixing eye at the null point which is in adduction. These patients will show a face turn towards the fixing eye, so the fixing eye is in adduction.

**Treatment:** MLN with esotropia and face turn is treated by correcting the strabismus to improve binocular fusion. If the patient has an accommodative component contributing to the esotropia then give the full plus spectacle correction. If there is even a small residual esotropia correct the esotropia. In patients without fusion potential, such as those with dense amblyopia, recess the MR muscle of the fixing eye in adduction to correct the face turn, and move the non-fixing eye to correct any residual or induced strabismus.

### Vertical and Torsional Head Posturing for Nystagmus

Similar principles regarding moving the null point to primary position applies to vertical head positions. The amount of surgery required to keep the eyes in primary position is large, up to 20 mm per eye, split between the superior rectus (SR) and inferior rectus (IR) muscles as reported by: Yang, Del Monte, and Archer from the University of Michigan.[1]

### Chin Elevation (Eyes Are Down)

A chin elevation is treated by moving the eyes up into primary position.

- 10° to 15°: recess IR 7 mm to 8 mm OU
- >15°: recess IR 7 mm to 8 mm and plicate or resect SR 7 mm OU

### Chin Depression (Eyes Are Up)

A chin depression is treated by moving the eyes down into primary position.

- 10° to 15°: recess SR 7 mm to 8 mm OU
- >15°: recess SR 7 mm to 8 mm and plicate or resect IR 5 mm to 6 mm OU

### Nystagmus with Head Tilt

Occasionally a compensatory head tilt is used to dampen the nystagmus. The strategy to correct the head tilt is to tort the eyes towards the head tilt.

Example: Head tilt to the right

Extort right eye
Intort left eye

Torsion can be induced by oblique muscle surgery such as Harada-Ito procedure to induce intorsion and tightening of the inferior oblique for extorsion. Unfortunately, these procedures also induce vertical and horizontal changes. Another method to induce torsion is by *transposing the vertical rectus muscles.*[2] Although this surgery may be indicated in rare cases, the author has never performed torsional surgery for nystagmus and head tilt.

- Extort right eye
  SR: nasal placement
  IR: temporal placement
- Intort left eye
  SR: temporal placement
  IR: nasal placement

*Nystagmus Without a Face Turn*

Some patients with nystagmus and no face turn will show visual improvement by four muscle retro-equatorial recessions. This procedure works best for motor nystagmus and only slightly, if at all, for sensory nystagmus such as in cases of albinism. Appropriate preoperative expectations are important as visual acuity improvement is modest at best, on an average only one line of improvement.[3] The author has found late occurrence of exotropia 3 to 5 years after symmetrical posterior equatorial recessions, so we now suggest recessing the MR muscle less than the LR muscle.

Surgery

Bilateral recessions MR 8.5 mm
Bilateral recessions LR 10.0 mm

# References

1. Yang MB, Pou-Vendrell CR, Archer SM, Martonyi EJ, Del Monte MA. Vertical rectus muscle surgery for nystagmus patients with vertical abnormal head posture. J AAPOS 2004;8:299–309.
2. von Noorden GK, Jenkins RH, Rosenbaum AL. Horizontal transposition of the vertical rectus muscles for treatment of ocular torticollis. J Pediatr Ophthalmol Strabismus 1993;30:8–14.
3. Helveston EM, Ellis FD, Plager DA. Large recession of the horizontal recti for treatment of nystagmus. Ophthalmology 1991;98:1302–1305.

# 7  Complex Strabismus

## Duane's Syndrome Type 1 (Esotropia)

*Clinical Features*

- Ipsilateral face turn
- Esotropia in primary position
- Abduction deficit
- Lid fissure narrowing in adduction, widening in abduction

*Etiology*

Pathophysiology is congenital agenesis of the sixth nerve nucleus and innervational misdirection of part of the medial rectus nerve to the lateral rectus muscle. This results in limited abduction and co-contraction of the medial and lateral recti on adduction. The co-contraction causes the globe to retract causing lid fissure narrowing on adduction. If the medial and lateral recti receive the same reciprocal innervation the eye will rest in primary position (equal). This results in a stand-off with equal medial and lateral forces so there is limited abduction and adduction or Duane's type 3 syndrome. In cases where the lateral rectus muscle receives more innervation an exotropia Duane's type 3 syndrome occurs. In most cases the medial rectus muscle gets most of the medial rectus nerve so the resting eye position is in adduction. This is esotropia Duane's syndrome type 1 (limited abduction, intact adduction). Duane's type 2 is characterized as good abduction with poor adduction. These cases are very rare (if they exist at all), and most cases are actually Duane's type 3. Synergistic divergence is a rare type of Duane's syndrome with abduction on attempted adduction. The lateral rectus muscle receives almost all the innervation from the medial rectus nerve, and there is agenesis of the sixth nerve nucleus.[1] Duane's syndrome is usually sporadic without systemic manifestations, however, it can be familial or associated with systemic disease (Goldenhar syndrome, Klippel-Feil syndrome, and intrauterine thalidomide exposure).

*Treatment*

The treatment of Duane's syndrome differs from a sixth nerve palsy because in Duane's syndrome the lateral rectus muscle is innervated, albeit by the medial rectus nerve. Thus there is a tonic lateral rectus muscle tone in Duane's syndrome, but not in sixth nerve palsy. The presence of lateral rectus tone is why a simple medial rectus recession works well to hold the

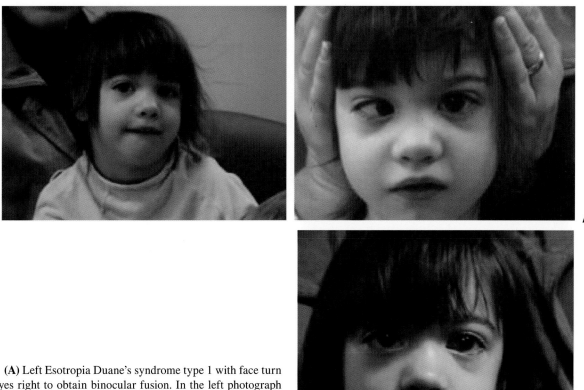

**FIGURE 7.1.** **(A)** Left Esotropia Duane's syndrome type 1 with face turn to the left, eyes right to obtain binocular fusion. In the left photograph note the left lid fissure is narrow when in adduction. Right photograph shows lid fissure widening on attempted abduction (poor abduction left eye). **(B)** Postoperative left medial rectus recession 6.0 mm showing no face turn and orthotropia in the primary position.

eye in primary position in patients with esotropia type 1 Duane's syndrome. Virtually all patients with esotropia type 1 Duane's syndrome will have a tight medial rectus muscle. Thus recession of the medial rectus muscle is of prime importance. The indication for surgery in esotropia Duane's syndrome type 1 is a significant face turn. Figure 7.1 shows pre- and postoperative photographs of a typical esotropia type 1 Duane's syndrome.

### Surgery for Type 1 Esotropia Duane's Syndrome (Author's Choice)

Procedure: Recess the ipsilateral medial rectus muscle.

- Moderate face turn (15° to 20°): 5.5 mm to 6.5 mm
- Large face turn (25° to 40°): 6.5 mm to 7.5 mm

For a residual esotropia and face turn after previous medial rectus recession, consider a re-recession ipsilateral MR of 3 mm to 4 mm. A residual esotropia usually persists if the previous MR recession was less than 6 mm, so one could re-recess the ipsilateral MR an additional 3 mm.

### Other Treatment Options

Some suggest using the transposition surgery as a primary procedure.[2] Disadvantages of the transposition surgery for Duane's syndrome include:

induced hypertropia (10% to 15%), high rate of undercorrection requiring a second operation, disruption of anterior ciliary circulation, and significantly more scarring than a simple medial rectus recession. The proposed advantage is improved abduction, but this has not been my experience.

Bilateral medial rectus recessions have been advocated to stimulate the Duane's eye to abduct through Hering's law of yoke muscles (medial and lateral recti are yoke muscles). However, recessing the contralateral medial rectus muscle does not improve abduction.[3] In Duane's syndrome the lateral rectus muscle is not innervated by the sixth nerve so Hering's law of yoke muscles does not apply.

## Duane's Syndrome Type 2

Duane's type 2 is identified as good abduction with poor adduction. These cases are very rare (if they exist at all), and most cases are actually Duane's type 3 (see Duane's type 3 for treatment).

## Duane's Syndrome Type 3 (Exotropia)

### Clinical Features

• Contralateral face turn
• Exotropia in primary position
• Abduction and adduction deficit (eye does not move much)
• Lid fissure narrowing in adduction, widening in abduction
• Upshoot and downshoot are frequent

### Treatment

• XT Duane's type 3 and contralateral face turn, perform an ipsilateral lateral rectus recession
• Duane's type 3 without a face turn (orthotropia in primary position), but severe co-contraction and lid fissure narrowing, perform an ipsilateral medial rectus recession and ipsilateral lateral rectus recession
• If an upshoot and downshoot are present add a Y-split procedure of the lateral rectus muscle (see later in this chapter, as well as Chapter 15).

## Duane's Syndrome with Upshoot and Downshoot

### Clinical Features

• Upshoot and downshoot on attempted adduction
• Usually Duane's type 3 with abduction and adduction deficit
• Lid fissure narrowing on adduction, widening on abduction

These patients have severe co-contraction and globe retraction, usually with marked lid fissure narrowing on attempted adduction. The upshoot or downshoot of the Duane's eye may be due to co-contraction of the lateral rectus muscle with slippage above and below the globe, or aberrant innervation of the vertical muscles with part of the medial rectus nerve.

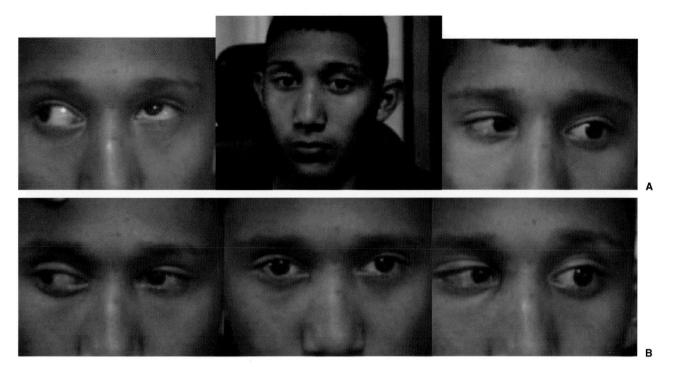

**FIGURE 7.2.** (A) Left exotropia Duane's type 3 syndrome with poor adduction and poor abduction. The center photograph shows a compensatory face turn to the right, eyes left. The left eye does not move horizontally as it is fixed in abduction. There is an upshoot of the left eye on attempted adduction. (B) Postoperative left lateral rectus recession 4 mm with Y-split. Note the improved adduction, head position, and absence of upshoot.

*Treatment*

- Duane's type 3 with upshoot or downshoot without a face turn (orthotropia in primary position), perform an ipsilateral medial rectus recession and ipsilateral lateral rectus recession with a Y-split of the recessed lateral rectus (see Chapter 15 for Y-split surgery). Note: Recession of the medial and lateral rectus muscles reduces the co-contraction, and the Y-split of the lateral rectus muscle reduces the upshoot and downshoot.[4]
- XT Duane's type 3 and contralateral face turn with an upshoot and downshoot, perform an ipsilateral lateral rectus recession 4 mm to 7 mm with Y-split (see Chapter 15 for Y-split surgery) (Figure 7.2).

## Synergistic Divergence

Synergistic divergence is characterized by abrupt abduction on attempted adduction—so both the eyes abduct on gaze away from the Duane's eye. Treatment consists of reducing the inappropriate abduction by eliminating ipsilateral lateral rectus function, and tightening the medial rectus muscle with a large resection. Lateral rectus function can be greatly reduced by total tenotomy or by suturing the lateral rectus muscle to the lateral orbital wall. Simultaneous removal of the inferior and superior oblique muscles has been suggested to further reduce abduction forces.[5]

## Congenital Fibrosis Syndrome

Congenital fibrosis syndromes (CFS) are associated with tight fibrotic muscles with the medial and inferior rectus most often involved. CFS is usually inherited as an autosomal dominant trait. There has been evidence that maldevelopment of the oculomotor (III), trochlear (IV), and abducens (VI) nuclei is associated with congenital fibrosis.[6] In rare cases there may be hypoplasia or **aplasia of the inferior rectus muscles** associated with muscle fibrosis without craniofacial dysostosis syndromes or neurofibromatosis.[7]

### Treatment

Treatment consists of recessing the tight muscles to improve ductions. If both the inferior rectus muscles are tight and there is a chin elevation recess both inferior recti. If there is a hypotropia perform asymmetric inferior rectus muscle recessions with a larger recession on the hypotropic side.[8] Esotropia can usually be treated by bilateral medial rectus recessions.

## A and V Patterns and Oblique Overaction

A and V Patterns (see Chapter 15)
Primary Inferior Oblique Overaction (see Chapter 17)
Primary Superior Oblique Overaction (see Chapter 19)

## Dissociated Strabismus Complex (DVD and DHD)

Dissociated vertical deviation (DVD) and dissociated horizontal deviation (DHD) occurs in approximately 40% of patients with infantile esotropia, usually presenting after 2 years of age. It can, however, occur primarily or secondarily with any disorder that disrupts normal binocular visual development. Two types of dissociated strabismus have been described: dissociated vertical deviation (DVD) and dissociated horizontal deviation (DHD), with DVD being the most commonly recognized form. Dissociated strabismus has three components: elevation, abduction, and extorsion. With DVD, the vertical component is predominant and with DHD, the horizontal component is predominant. Dissociated strabismus is typically latent and is manifest when one eye is occluded for several seconds. It can also become manifest spontaneously, often occurring when the patient is fatigued or is daydreaming.

DVD is characterized by a slow drift of one eye up and out with slight extorsion. It is almost always bilateral but is often asymmetric. DVD can be distinguished from a true hypertropia by the lack of a corresponding hypotropia in the contralateral eye when the ipsilateral hypertropic eye returns to primary position (Figure 7.3).

DHD has a similar appearance to consecutive exotropia, with an eye that will intermittently drift outward especially when the child is tired or daydreaming. In unilateral cases, covering the DHD eye induces an exo-drift, but there is no drift when the fellow eye is covered. DHD can be unilateral, bilateral or asymmetric. In cases where there is a small residual esotropia plus a unilateral DHD, alternate cover testing will disclose an exo-shift (inward movement) from the DHD eye, while the fellow eye will

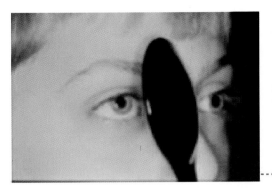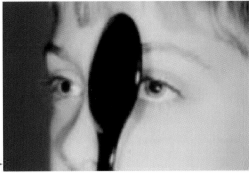

FIGURE 7.3. Shows bilateral DVD with a right hypertropia with the right eye covered and a left hypertropia with the left eye covered.

show an eso-shift (outward movement). If the DHD is larger than 10 to 15 PD, it can be symptomatic and may need surgery.

*Treatment*

Surgery is indicated if the deviation is obvious and bothersome to the patient or parents, or if the deviation is increasing in frequency.

- **DHD:** Ipsilateral lateral rectus recession (usually 4 mm to 6 mm)
- **DVD:** Ipsilateral large superior rectus recession between 5 mm and 8 mm (fixed suture technique)
  Most cases require bilateral surgery; if the DVD is asymmetric, then perform asymmetric superior rectus recessions. Patients with amblyopia ≥2 lines will not fixate with the amblyopic eye and, in these cases, unilateral surgery is indicated (a superior rectus muscle recession of the amblyopic eye).
- **DVD + Inferior Oblique Overaction:** DVD and inferior oblique overaction often coexist. In these cases, an inferior oblique anteriorization procedure is indicated as it will correct both the inferior oblique overaction and DVD. Avoid combining inferior oblique anteriorization and superior rectus recession as this will significantly limit up gaze. Severe DVD and mild inferior oblique overaction can be treated with a small inferior oblique recession and a superior rectus recession but, in most cases, an inferior oblique anteriorization will be sufficient.

## Thyroid Strabismus

Strabismus associated with thyroid eye disease occurs as inflamed muscles change to become fibrotic and stiff. All the extraocular muscles are affected, but the inferior and medial rectus muscles are most severely involved. Asymmetric inferior rectus fibrosis will cause a hypotropia with limited elevation of both eyes, worse on the side of the hypotropic eye. Fibrosis of the medial rectus muscles results in an esotropia. A combination of hypotropia and esotropia commonly occurs. Involvement of the lateral rectus muscle is uncommon, however, if there is an exotropia one must rule out a history of prior orbital decompression or co-existent myasthenia gravis. Surgery should be performed only after the acute inflammatory phase subsides, and the angle of strabismus is stable.

The basic surgical strategy is to recess the tight muscles that limit ductions; avoid resections. There is a high rate of late overcorrection after strabismus surgery for thyroid related eye disease. Hudson and Feldon reported that 50% of inferior rectus recessions had a late overcorrection occurring 4 to 8 weeks after surgery.[9] The most likely explanation is a stretched insertion scar or dehiscence, which occurs as the suture dissolves.[10]

Adjustable sutures and the hang-back technique may contribute to poor scleral fixation and an increased risk of stretched scar. If bilateral IR recessions are done, the late overcorrection is not clinically as obvious because both sides slip. These patients often develop superior oblique overaction, A pattern, and a large exotropia in down gaze. Recent literature has emphasized good results using a fixed suture technique rather than adjustable sutures.[11] Many (yes, I am in this group) now use nonabsorbable (5-0 Mersilene) sutures and avoid adjustable sutures when performing strabismus surgery for thyroid eye disease.

### Treatment

### Hypotropia (Tight Inferior Rectus Muscle)

For a unilateral hypotropia in the primary position and good motility of the fellow eye, recess the ipsilateral inferior rectus muscle. Plan on correcting about 3 PD of vertical deviation for every 1.0 mm of inferior rectus recession. If both inferior rectus muscles are tight, then do bilateral inferior rectus recessions, doing more on the hypotropic eye. Bilateral inferior rectus recessions reduce the problem of late overcorrection but increase the risk of late postoperative A pattern and SO overaction (weak IR OU).

- Hypotropia ≤ 15 PD: recess ipsilateral inferior rectus muscle
- Hypotropia >15 PD: recess ipsilateral inferior rectus muscle and contralateral superior rectus muscle

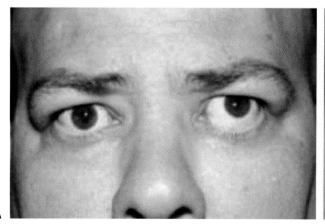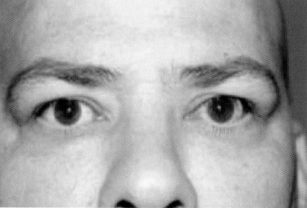

**FIGURE 7.4. (A)** Stretched scar with slipped IR and MR. Patient with thyroid strabismus and previous left inferior and medial rectus recession. Note the consecutive exotropia, left hypertropia, and left lower lid retraction. The inferior and medial rectus muscles have slipped posteriorly due to a stretched scar. Note that the slipped inferior rectus is responsible for the lower lid retraction. The treatment is to advance the inferior and medial rectus muscles using a non-absorbable suture. **(B)** Postoperative advancement of slipped IR and MR in the left eye with a non-absorbable suture. Note the excellent alignment, improved ductions, and good lower lid position of the left eye.

# Brown's Syndrome

*Clinical Features*

1. Deficient elevation in adduction
2. Minimal or less deficient elevation in abduction
3. Positive forced ductions up and in
4. Minimal or no superior oblique overaction
5. Y-pattern or no pattern

Brown's syndrome should be divided into congenital and acquired forms.

*Congenital Brown's Syndrome*

Congenital Brown's Syndrome is a constant, stable condition that rarely resolves spontaneously. Surgery may be required in these cases. The etiology seems to be an inelastic or stiff superior oblique muscle tendon complex.[12]

## Indications for Surgery

Surgical indications include a chin elevation, face turn, or severe limitation of elevation in adduction.

## Surgical Procedure

A controlled elongation of the superior oblique (SO) tendon is the best approach, using either the superior oblique tendon silicone expander (Wright procedure) or the split tendon elongation (see Chapter 19).

## Complications of Surgery

**Undercorrection:** A mild residual limitation of elevation in adduction is a good result and should be left alone. Even an immediate severe undercorrection will usually show improvement over weeks to several months. If there is a significant undercorrection consider missed posterior SO tendon fibers. Another possibility is that the limitation of elevation is not caused by a tight SO tendon as there are non-SO tendon related causes of Brown's syndrome. Bhola et al. used high resolution MRI to identify alternative etiologies for presumed tight SO tendon Brown's syndrome, including an infra-placed LR muscle pulley in adduction.[13] These alternative causes of Brown's syndrome helps explain the basis for occasional undercorrections.

Superior oblique tenotomy or tenectomy for Brown's syndrome results in a consecutive SO palsy in more than 50% of cases. The use of graded elongation procedures such as the Wright's silicone tendon expander and the split tendon elongation procedure have reduced the incidence to less than 10%.[12] Superior oblique surgery is difficult and requires a delicate and careful approach. Complications of superior oblique surgery are covered in Chapter 19.

*Acquired Brown's Syndrome*

## Causes

| | |
|---|---|
| Sinusitis | Sinus surgery |
| Superior oblique tuck | Orbital trauma |

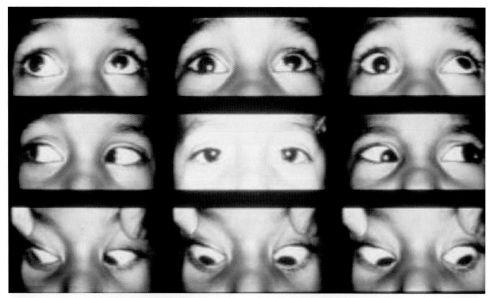

A

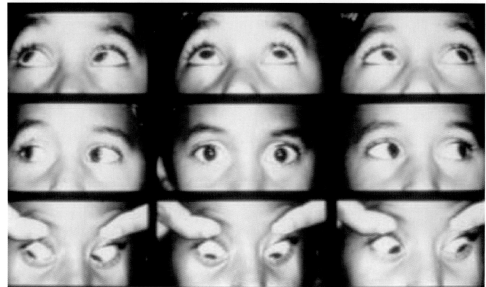

B

FIGURE 7.5. (A) shows a preoperative composite photograph of a patient with a right congenital Brown's syndrome. Notice the limitation of elevation that is worse in adduction (but present in abduction) right eye, the presence of a V-pattern, and lack of superior oblique overaction. (B) shows a postoperative composite photograph after a 6.0mm Wright's silicone tendon expander procedure was done, and it demonstrates essentially normal versions.

Retinal surgery                 Glaucoma implants
Thyroid disease                 Blepharoplasty
Trochlear bursitis              JRA, adult RA
Lupus                           Scleroderma
Stenosing tenosynovitis

Patients with acquired Brown's Syndrome should be worked up with an MRI scan to rule out orbital pathology. This form is best treated conservatively without surgery, as many will resolve spontaneously. Inflammatory Brown's syndrome, a type of acquired Brown's syndrome, is treated with oral antiinflammatory medications, such as ibuprofen, or a local injection of corticosteroids. Noninflammatory acquired Brown's syndrome that remains constant for years, can be treated surgically. Some of these cases of acquired Brown's syndrome can show improvement after several years of observation.

Sinusitis is probably an important cause of acquired Brown's syndrome, and should be treated if present. Trauma to the area of the trochlea can cause a Brown's syndrome, but there is often a coexisting ipsilateral superior oblique paresis. These cases are difficult to manage as surgery on the trochlea can lead to more scarring and increase restriction, and a superior oblique weakening procedure will make a superior oblique paresis worse.

### Canine Tooth Syndrome

Trauma to the trochlear area can cause scarring that restricts the movement of the superior oblique tendon. This produces both a Brown's syndrome (restriction) and a superior oblique paresis. These cases are difficult to manage as surgery to try to remove scarring can lead to more scarring and increase restriction. Superior oblique weakening procedures only worsen the superior oblique paresis.

### Double Elevator Palsy (Monocular Elevation Deficit Syndrome)

*Clinical Features*

- Elevation deficit similar or worse in abduction vs. adduction
- No superior oblique overaction
- Forced ductions show tight inferior rectus in 70% of cases

Double elevator palsy is a limited elevation of one eye across the board in adduction and abduction. The term "double elevator" implies paresis of the superior rectus and inferior oblique muscle. This is, however, a misnomer as the deficient elevation is due to restriction from a tight inferior rectus in 70% of the cases. Double elevator palsy may be mistaken for Brown's syndrome, but remember that in Brown's syndrome, the limited elevation is worse in adduction than in abduction. The condition presents clinically as a hypotropia; a chin elevation and ptosis are often present. True ptosis due to levator weakness is present in 50% to 60% of cases, while pseudoptosis may occur in almost all patients with a large hypotropia when fixating with the sound eye. Other abnormal innervational conditions associated with double elevator palsy include jaw-winking, Duane's syndrome, and other misdirection strabismus syndromes.

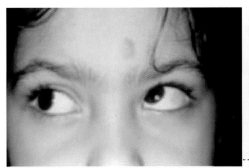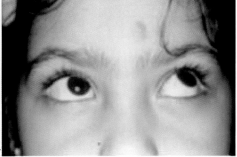

**FIGURE 7.6.** A right double elevator palsy caused by a paretic superior rectus muscle. Note the limited elevation is worse in abduction (*left*) compared to elevation in adduction (*right*).

*Treatment*

Surgery is indicated if there is a chin elevation due to a vertical strabismus in primary gaze. If a good up gaze saccade is seen clinically, and forced ductions show a tight inferior rectus muscle, then a simple recession of the inferior rectus muscle is indicated. If up gaze saccades are deficient, the cause of the elevation deficit is a weak superior rectus muscle, and a vertical transposition procedure is indicated. I prefer the vertical Hummelsheim with the Foster modification as it spares the anterior ciliary vessels and it is a strong procedure that works well. The vertical Hummelsheim consists of transposing half the medial rectus muscle and half the lateral rectus muscle superiorly toward the superior rectus muscle (see Chapter 16).

### Tight Inferior Rectus Muscle, with Good Superior Rectus Muscle Function

- Recess ipsilateral inferior rectus muscle (usually around 6 mm).

### Superior Rectus Muscle Palsy

- Recess ipsilateral inferior rectus muscle and split tendon transfer of one-half medial rectus and one-half lateral rectus to the superior rectus muscle (vertical Hummelsheim) with the Foster modification (see Chapters 15 and 16).

## Orbital Floor Fracture

Restrictive strabismus in orbital floor fractures is due to entrapment of orbital fat and sometimes, the inferior rectus muscle into the fracture. This leads to scarring of the inferior rectus muscle to the fractured floor, causing restriction of elevation and positive forced ductions. Often there will also be limited depression that can persist even after the floor fracture has been repaired. The cause of the limited depression is probably scarring of the inferior rectus muscle to the orbital floor so the inferior rectus muscle can not transmit its full pull to the globe. Limited depression of the eye associated with a floor fracture is rarely due to an inferior rectus palsy. Signs of a blow-out fracture include vertical diplopia, enophthalmos, and hypoesthesia of the cheek and upper gum on the affected side. Strabismus surgery is indicated if diplopia persists for 6 to 8 weeks after repair of the floor fracture.

*Tight Inferior Rectus, Restricted Elevation*

Floor fracture with inferior rectus restriction can cause limited elevation with a hypertropia that increases in up gaze. The first line of treatment is to repair the floor fracture, but a residual restriction may persist. If there is a hypertropia in all vertical gaze positions, an ipsilateral inferior rectus recession is indicated. Often, however, the eyes are aligned in down gaze with a hypertropia in up gaze. Examples 7.1 and 7.2 show typical patterns of strabismus associated with a left floor fracture after repair.

---

*Example 7.1. Hypertropia after Left Floor Fracture and Repair*

Ductions Right eye: full, Left eye: limitation of elevation −1

| | |
|---|---|
| Up gaze | RHT 18 PD |
| Primary | RHT 10 PD |
| Down gaze | RHT 4 PD |

**Surgical Strategy:** There is a tight left inferior rectus muscle with a right hypertropia in all fields of gaze, worse in up gaze. Recessing the left inferior rectus will release the restriction and improve the alignment. There might be a small residual right hypertropia in up gaze and a small consecutive left hypertropia in down gaze but the deviation will be much improved.

---

*Example 7.2. Hypertropia Up Gaze after Left Floor Fracture and Repair*

Ductions Right eye: full, Left eye: limitation of elevation

| | |
|---|---|
| Up gaze | RHT 18 PD |
| Primary | RHT 5 PD |
| Down gaze | Orthotropia |

**Surgical Strategy:** There is a tight left inferior rectus muscle but little hypertropia in primary and orthotropia in down gaze. Recessing the inferior rectus muscle enough to improve up gaze will induce a left hypertropia in primary and down gaze. Remember a recession has its greatest effect toward the recessed muscle. A useful strategy is to perform bilateral inferior rectus recessions and a contralateral (right) superior rectus recession, depending on the hypertropia in primary position. This preserves alignment in primary and down gaze while reducing the hypertropia in primary position and up gaze (see Chapter 6).

---

*Pseudo Inferior Rectus Palsy, Limited Depression*

An unusual, but important, strabismus after floor fracture is limited depression that can persist even after the floor fracture has been repaired. The cause of the limited depression is probably the inferior rectus being tethered by inferior scarring, so the inferior rectus muscle can not transmit its full pull to the globe. As the eye rotates down, the anterior muscle slack builds up, reducing the muscle's function. There is typically a good saccadic eye movement from up gaze to primary position, but slow eye movement from primary position to down gaze. The intact saccadic movements from up gaze to primary position indicate good inferior rectus function.

---

*Example 7.3.  Limited Depression after a Left Floor Fracture and Repair*

Ductions Right eye: full, Left eye: limitation of depression −1

| | |
|---|---|
| Up gaze | Orthotropia |
| Primary | LHT 9 PD |
| Down gaze | LHT 18 PD |

**Surgical Strategy:** Plication of the ipsilateral inferior rectus muscle (small 2.5 mm to 3.5 mm) and contralateral inferior rectus muscle recession. The plication is important as it removes the anterior muscle slack, improving down gaze.

---

This is almost never a true inferior rectus palsy. Below is the typical pattern of strabismus associated with a left floor fracture and pseudoinferior rectus palsy.

## Strabismus Associated with Local Anesthetic Injection

Injection of a local anesthetic such as lidocaine or mepivacaine, into an extraocular muscle, can change the muscle's function and cause strabismus. Retrobulbar or peribulbar anesthetic injections for a variety of ophthalmic procedures such as cataract surgery or retinal detachment surgery may inadvertently result in an intramuscular injection. With the advent of topical anesthesia for cataract surgery, the incidence of strabismus after cataract surgery has dropped significantly. The inferior rectus (usually left eye–right handed surgeon) is most frequently involved, but all muscles are vulnerable, including the superior rectus muscle.

Initially the injected muscle is paretic for several days causing a hypertropia in the case of the inferior rectus muscle. Then, over a week or two, the muscle undergoes fibrosis. This intramuscular fibrosis tightens the muscle, but also can cause the muscle to overact—actually gain strength. Some theorize that increased Z band overlap is a cause of increased muscle strength. In the case of the inferior rectus muscle, the hypertropia changes over a few weeks to a hypotropia. The inferior rectus muscle overacts, and the hypotropia will be greatest in down gaze. It is hypothesized that the overaction is due to intramuscular fibrosis changing the length tendon curve, increasing muscle strength. Infrequently, the inferior rectus will simply be tight from the fibrosis, and in these cases the hypotropia is greater in up gaze.

Initially follow the patient to see if the deviation spontaneously improves. If after 6 weeks a significant deviation persists, then consider strabismus surgery. The surgical treatment is relatively simple and highly effective—a recession of the overacting muscle. Because recessions have their greatest weakening effect in the field of action of the recessed muscle, a simple recession works beautifully to correct the overacting muscle and correct the incomitance (see Example 7.4).

*Example 7.4. 60 year old had a retrobulbar injection of lidocaine and mepivacaine left eye for cataract surgery. Immediately after cataract surgery diplopia was noted, associated with a left hypertropia which increased in down gaze. The left inferior rectus showed significant underaction. Two weeks later the deviation reversed and a right hypertropia increasing in down gaze was measured. This deviation persisted and is shown below.*

Deviation 8 weeks after cataract surgery

Ductions: limitation of elevation left eye −1
  Up gaze:          RHT 7 PD
  Primary:          RHT 12 PD
  Down gaze:       RHT 18 PD

**Surgical Strategy:** The left inferior rectus is overacting as the hypertropia is greatest in down gaze. Recess the overacting left inferior rectus muscle 4 mm to 5 mm as we tend to get about 3 PD for every 1 mm vertical rectus muscle recession. Since the inferior rectus recession has its greatest weakening effect in down gaze the surgery will nicely correct the vertical incomitance.

## High Myopia and Esotropia

### Bilateral Myopia and Esotropia

Progressive high myopia (>10.00 PD) can cause an acquired esotropia with or without a hypotropia. Bilateral high myopia, as seen in example of Figure 7.7, can cause a large angle esotropia with limited abduction. The cause is axial length elongation in the superior temporal direction, that displaces the lateral rectus muscle inferiorly, reducing its abduction function thus causing an esotropia. The ectopic locations of the muscles can be seen with orbital MRI. One treatment I have found effective is to perform large medial rectus muscle recessions and to transpose the lateral rectus muscle superiorly by suturing them to the sclera at the equator. Usually the sclera at the equator is thick enough to allow safe needle passes.

### Heavy Eye Syndrome

High myopia (>−20.00) with severe axial length elongation that causes an esotropia, and hypotropia, with limited abduction and elevation, is termed heavy eye syndrome (Figure 7.8). Superior temporal expansion of the globe displaces the lateral rectus muscle inferiorly and the superior rectus muscle nasally (Figure 7.8). This muscle displacement changes the vector of forces of the muscles. The lateral rectus muscle loses its abduction function and becomes a depressor, while the superior rectus muscle changes from an elevator to an adductor. The treatment of the heavy eye syndrome (esotropia and hypotropia) is to move the displaced muscles back to their appropriate location.[14] The lateral rectus muscle is transposed superiorly, and the superior rectus muscle temporally and united at the equator with a non-absorbable suture like a Jensen transposition (see Chapter 16). The

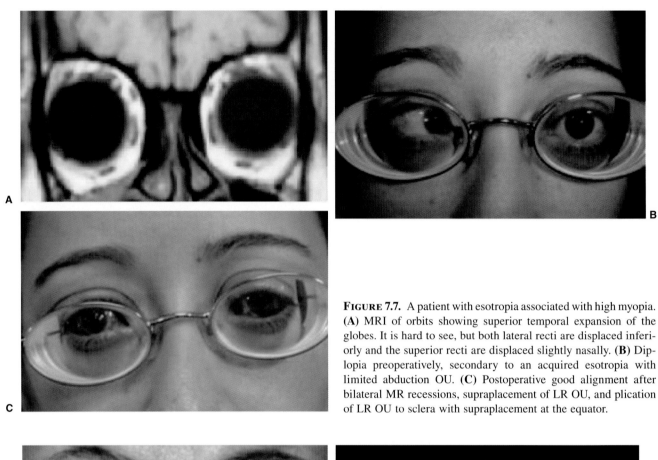

**FIGURE 7.7.** A patient with esotropia associated with high myopia. **(A)** MRI of orbits showing superior temporal expansion of the globes. It is hard to see, but both lateral recti are displaced inferiorly and the superior recti are displaced slightly nasally. **(B)** Diplopia preoperatively, secondary to an acquired esotropia with limited abduction OU. **(C)** Postoperative good alignment after bilateral MR recessions, supraplacement of LR OU, and plication of LR OU to sclera with supraplacement at the equator.

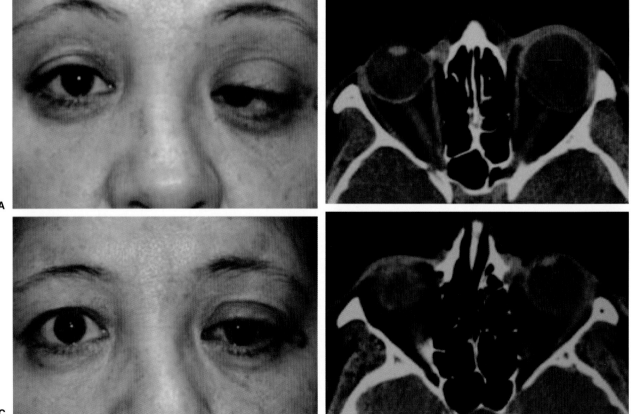

**FIGURE 7.8.** **(A)** Heavy eye syndrome with left eye fixed in adduction and depression (limitation of abduction −4 and poor elevation left eye). **(B)** CT scan: *Left* photograph shows posterior staphyloma pushing the lateral rectus down out of view. *Right* scan of a lower cut shows lateral rectus that is displaced inferiorly. **(C)** Postoperative left medial rectus recession and union of the superior rectus and lateral rectus muscles at the equator. There is a small residual left hypotropia.

suture is passed 14 mm posterior to the insertion, and through one half width of each muscle as described by Yokoyama. In addition, perform a medial rectus recession, as the medial rectus will be tight.

## References

1. Kim JH, Hwang JM. Hypoplastic oculomotor nerve and absent abducens nerve in congenital fibrosis syndrome and synergistic divergence with magnetic resonance imaging. Ophthalmology 2005;112:728–732.
2. Velez FG, Foster RS, MD. Rosenbaum A. Vertical rectus muscle augmented transposition in Duane Syndrome. J AAPOS 2001;5:105–113.
3. Greenberg MF, Pollard Z. Poor results after recession of both medial rectus muscles in unilateral small-angle Duane's Syndrome Type I. J AAPOS 2003;7:142–145.
4. Raina J, Wright KW, Lin MM, McVey JH. Effectiveness of lateral rectus Y-split surgery for correcting the upshoot and downshoot in Duane's retraction syndrome. Type III. Binocular Vision Strabismus 1997;12:233–238.
5. Mohan K, Gupta R, Sharma A, Gupta A. Treatment of congenital adduction palsy with synergistic divergence. J Pediatr Ophthalmol Strabismus 1998;35:149–152. Erratum in: J Pediatr Ophthalmol Strabismus 1998;35:226.
6. Demer JL, Clark RA, Engle EC. Magnetic resonance imaging evidence for widespread orbital dysinnervation in congenital fibrosis of extraocular muscles due to mutations in KIF21A. Invest Ophthalmol Vis Sci 2005;46:530–539.
7. Pimenides D, Young S, Minty I, Spratt J, Tiffin PA. Familial aplasia of the inferior rectus muscles. J Pediatr Ophthalmol Strabismus 2005;42:222–227.
8  Yazdani A, Traboulsi EI. Classification and surgical management of patients with familial and sporadic forms of congenital fibrosis of the extraocular muscles. Ophthalmology 2004;111:1035–1042.
9. Hudson HL, Feldon SE, Gilbert J. Late overcorrection of hypotropia in Graves ophthalmopathy. Predictive factors. Ophthalmology 1992;99:356–360.
10. Ludwig I. Scar remodeling after strabismus surgery. Trans Am Ophthalmol Soc 1999;97:583–651.
11. Gilbert J, Dailey RA, Christensen LE. Characteristics and outcomes of strabismus surgery after orbital decompression for thyroid eye disease. J AAPOS 2005;9:26–30.
12. Wright KW. Brown's syndrome: diagnosis and management. Trans Am Ophthalmol Soc 1999;97:1023–1109.
13. Bhola R, Rosenbaum AL, Ortube MC, Demer JL. High-resolution magnetic resonance imaging demonstrates varied anatomic abnormalities in Brown syndrome. J AAPOS 2005;9:438–448.
14. Yokoyama T, et al. Treatment of progressive esotropia caused by high myopia— A new surgical procedure based on its pathogenesis. Transaction of the 27th meeting, European Strabismological Association, Italy, June 2001, de Faber, J.T.H.N. (ed). Swets & Zeitlinger Publishers, Lisse, 2002; pp 145–158.

# 8 Cranial Nerve Palsies

## Superior Oblique Palsy

### Clinical Features

The clinical features of superior oblique paresis vary widely depending on the type. Common features include an ipsilateral hypertropia that increases on contralateral gaze, and a positive head tilt test with the hypertropia increasing on head tilt to the side of the hypertropia. Congenital superior oblique paresis is commonly associated with ipsilateral inferior oblique overaction and relatively less superior oblique underaction. Acquired superior oblique paresis, on the other hand, has relatively normal versions, minimal inferior oblique overaction, but significant extorsional diplopia. The head tilt test can help differentiate primary inferior oblique overaction from inferior oblique overaction secondary to superior oblique paresis. A positive head tilt test indicates a superior oblique paresis and a negative head tilt test suggests primary inferior oblique overaction.

### Parks Three-Step Test

The Parks three-step test is used in patients with a hypertropia, to help diagnose if a vertical muscle is paretic and to identify the paretic muscle. The head tilt test is a crucial part of the test. If the head tilt reveals a change of more than 5 PD on tilt from one side to the opposite side, it is considered a positive test and indicates the strong possibility of a vertical muscle palsy. The paretic muscle is identified by completing the Parks three-step test (see Table 8.1). For example, a patient presents with a left hypertropia that increases in right gaze and increases on left head tilt (Figure 8.1). The highlighted muscles in Table 8.1 show the process of elimination (left to right) to identify the paretic muscle: left superior oblique (LSO). A positive head tilt test is not pathognomonic of a vertical muscle palsy. Both dissociated vertical deviation, and a small hypertropia associated with intermittent exotropia, can have positive head tilt tests. The head tilt test is only applicable to a single paretic vertical muscle, as multiple paretic muscles or the presence of restrictive strabismus make the test unreliable.

### Head Tilt Test Made Easy

Because of the complexity of the three-step test, it is difficult to do it in your mind without a paper and pencil and at least one textbook on strabismus. A trick that simplifies the three-step test is to consider the head tilt first. If the hypertropia increases on head tilt to the side of the hypertropia then an oblique muscle is paretic. A hypertropia that increases on head tilt

**TABLE 8.1.** Parks Three-Step Test

| First step<br>hyper in<br>primary position | | Second step<br>hyper increases<br>in gaze | | Third step<br>hyper increases<br>with head tilt |
|---|---|---|---|---|
| **RHT** | RSO<br>RIR<br><br>LSR<br>LIO | **R** | RIR<br><br>LIO | **R** = LIO<br>**L** = RIR |
| | | **L** | RSO<br><br>LSR | **R** = RSO<br>**L** = LSR |
| **LHT** | **RSR**<br>**RIO**<br><br>**LSO**<br>**LIR** | **R** | **RSR**<br><br>**LSO** | **R** = RSR<br>**L = LSO** |
| | | **L** | RIO<br><br>LIR | **R** = LIR<br>**L** = RIO |

to the opposite side of the hypertropia is caused by a paretic vertical rectus muscle. This quickly narrows the field of possibilities. For example, a left hypertropia that increases on head tilt to the left (same side as the hypertropia) indicates a paretic oblique muscle either LSO or RIO. If the left hypertropia increases in right gaze it is a paretic LSO. If the left hypertropia increases in left gaze it is a RIO palsy.

*Unilateral versus Bilateral Superior Oblique Paresis*

Signs of unilateral and bilateral superior oblique paresis are listed in Table 8.2. A unilateral superior oblique palsy typically has a significant hypertropia in the primary position that increases to the opposite gaze and with tilt to the side of the hypertropia. Signs of a bilateral superior oblique

**TABLE 8.2.** Unilateral versus Bilateral Superior Oblique Paresis

| Clinical Sign | Unilateral | Bilateral |
|---|---|---|
| Superior oblique underaction | Ipsilateral underaction | Bilateral underaction |
| Inferior oblique overaction | Ipsilateral overaction | Bilateral overaction |
| V-pattern | Less than 10 PD | Greater than 10 PD |
| Hypertropia | Greater than 5 PD | Less than 5 PD (except asymmetric paresis) |
| Head tilt test | Increasing hyper on ipsilateral head tilt | Positive head tilt test to both sides (RHT tilt right and LHT tilt left) |
| Objective torsion on fundus exam | Ipsilateral | Bilateral |
| Extorsion on double Maddox rod test | Less than 10° (congenital; usually do not have subjective extorsion) | Greater than 10° (congenital; usually do not have subjective extorsion) |

palsy include small or no hypertropia in the primary position, reversing hypertropias in side gaze, and head tilt. There is a right hypertropia on tilt right and left hypertropia on tilt left, and a right hypertropia in left gaze, and a left hypertropia in right gaze. The presence of a V-pattern and bilateral extorsion on fundus exam further suggest bilateral involvement.

An asymmetric bilateral superior oblique paresis can look like a unilateral superior oblique paresis and is termed masked bilateral superior oblique paresis. A masked bilateral paresis should be suspected if there is even trace inferior oblique overaction of the opposite eye. Also, if there is a large hypertropia in the primary position that precipitously diminishes on gaze to the same side of the hypertropia, consider a masked bilateral superior oblique paresis. For example, a patient has a left superior oblique palsy with a LHT 20 PD in the primary position that diminishes to LHT 2 PD in left gaze, and trace right inferior oblique overaction (Figure 8.1).

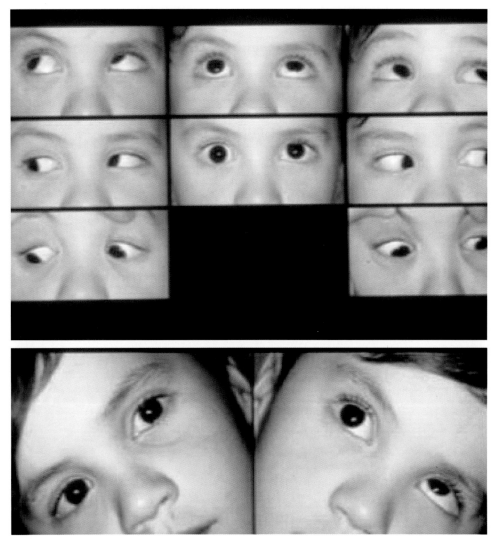

Right gaze                          Primary position                     Left gaze
LHT 30 PD                          LHT 20 PD                            LHT 2 PD
Head tilt right—LHT 3 PD      Head tilt left—LHT 25 PD

**FIGURE 8.1.** Masked bilateral superior oblique palsy.

This indicates that the right superior oblique is also paretic with right inferior oblique overaction reducing the left hypertropia in left gaze. Surgery for a unilateral superior oblique palsy can unmask a masked bilateral superior oblique paresis with postoperative overaction of the contralateral inferior oblique muscle.

### Congenital Superior Oblique Palsy

The cause of congenital superior oblique palsy is unknown. In some cases the superior oblique paresis is associated with a lax tendon and, rarely, an absent superior oblique tendon. The Indiana group suggests performing an exaggerated forced duction test of the superior oblique tendon at the beginning of surgery to see if the tendon is lax or absent.[1]

## Clinical Features

Patients with congenital superior oblique paresis adopt a compensatory head tilt opposite the side of the palsy to minimize the deviation and establish binocular fusion. Facial asymmetry is commonly present and may be the result of chronic head tilt. There is usually a large hypertropia in the primary position and a significant inferior oblique overaction, usually with relatively less superior oblique underaction. Although the paresis is present at birth, the first clinical signs of congenital superior oblique paresis often present in late childhood or even adulthood. Patients with congenital superior oblique paresis develop large vertical fusional amplitudes and fuse large hypertropias up to 35 PD. The presence of large vertical fusion amplitudes is an important clinical sign that the hyperdeviation is long standing, rather than acquired, and is suggestive of a congenital superior oblique palsy. Fusional control weakens over time, resulting in a deviation that becomes manifest in later life. Review of family photographs will often document a long standing head tilt opposite to the side of the hypertropia, indicating a congenital rather than an acquired superior oblique palsy.

Patients with congenital superior oblique paresis typically have good stereopsis and manifest the hyperdeviation intermittently when they are fatigued. Even though patients with congenital superior oblique paresis typically have high-grade stereopsis, most have the ability to suppress avoiding diplopia. Some patients will complain of diplopia, but usually not torsional, although they have objective extorsion on indirect ophthalmoscopy.

## Indications for Surgery

Surgery is indicated for a significant head tilt, a hypertropia causing asthenopia, and symptomatic diplopia. The timing of surgery is controversial. Some suggest early surgery, even in infancy, to prevent secondary facial asymmetry, while others advocate waiting until 2 to 3 years of age. Advocates for late surgery reason that strabismus measurements are more reliable and binocular function is more mature and stable after infancy. There is no good evidence to clearly choose. The author's advice is to wait until 2 years of age as long as the head tilt is mild and binocular fusion is maintained. In cases of severe head tilt, or if binocular fusion is compromised, early surgery is indicated.

### Tight Superior Rectus Muscle: "Jampolsky Syndrome"

Patients with a long-standing congenital superior oblique palsy and a large hypertropia may develop secondary contracture of the ipsilateral superior rectus muscle. This will cause a hypertropia in both right and left gaze, with pseudo-overaction of the contralateral superior oblique muscle. This occurs as the ipsilateral superior rectus is tight, limiting depression more in abduction, and as shown by Hering's law, induces contralateral superior oblique overaction. The hypertropia is greater in down gaze. Treatment is to consider adding an ipsilateral superior rectus recession to the treatment plan. Avoid weakening the contralateral superior oblique muscle.

### Prism Treatment

Prisms are usually of limited value because of the incomitance. In some older adults, prisms can be used to help control the deviation. If prisms are used, undercorrect the deviation to stimulate vertical fusion amplitudes.

### Surgical Treatment

The surgical plan depends on the pattern of the strabismus. In general, most types of congenital superior oblique palsy can be treated by the following formulas:

Unilateral
- Hypertropia <18 PD: Graded anteriorization ipsilateral inferior oblique muscle
- Hypertropia >18 PD: Graded anteriorization ipsilateral inferior oblique muscle, and contralateral inferior rectus recession (if there is a significant hyper in down gaze)

Bilateral
- Hypertropia <8 PD: Bilateral inferior oblique graded anteriorization with greater anteriorization on the hypertropic side

Masked bilateral (Figure 8.1)
- Ipsilateral inferior oblique muscle anteriorization and contralateral inferior rectus recession plus contralateral inferior oblique recession

Lax superior oblique tendon
- Superior oblique tuck has been suggested for patients with congenital superior oblique paresis secondary to a congenitally lax superior oblique tendon.[1] The tuck, however, has the common complication of iatrogenic Brown's syndrome and is reserved for rare cases of severe superior oblique laxity. Tendon tucking is reserved for extremely lax superior oblique tendon

Residual head tilt after inferior oblique weakening procedure
- Harada-Ito procedure opposite side to the head tilt

### Traumatic Superior Oblique Paresis

Traumatic superior oblique paresis is usually associated with severe closed head trauma, loss of consciousness, and cerebral concussion. Since the two trochlear nerves exit the mid brain together only a few millimeters apart, the nerve trauma is almost always bilateral, but the paresis may be quite asymmetrical. Classically, there is a small, or no, hypertropia in the primary position, a right hypertropia on tilt right and in left gaze, and a left hypertropia on tilt left and in right gaze. There is a V pattern-arrow type with an esotropia in down gaze, and extorsion worse in down gaze. Since the strabismus is acquired, patients will complain of torsional, vertical, and horizontal diplopia that increases in down gaze. Torsional diplopia associated with head trauma is a superior oblique palsy until proven otherwise.

### Indications for Surgery

Observe conservatively for at least 6 months taking serial measurements of the deviation. If, after 6 months of observation, the superior oblique paresis persists with symptomatic diplopia, surgery should be considered (see surgery strategies later in this chapter). Prism glasses are usually not useful because of the torsion and incomitance of the deviation.

### Surgical Treatment

The surgical plan for most traumatic bilateral superior oblique paresis with extorsion, and esotropia >8 to 10 PD in down gaze but no significant hypertropia in the primary position:

- Bilateral Harada-Ito Procedure: If a small hyperdeviation is present, do an asymmetric Harada-Ito by securing a larger width of the superior oblique tendon and increasing the tightening on the side of the hypertropia, plus
- Bilateral medial rectus recessions (small) with infraplacement one-half tendon width.

### Other Causes of Superior Oblique Paresis

The majority of superior oblique paresis are either congenital or traumatic, but other causes include vascular disease, multiple sclerosis, intracranial neoplasm, herpes zoster ophthalmicus, diabetes mellitus and associated mononeuropathy, and iatrogenic results after superior oblique tenotomy. If no specific cause of an acquired superior oblique paresis can be found, a neurological work-up including neuroimaging should be performed.

### General Treatment Guidelines for Superior Oblique Paresis

The treatment of superior oblique paresis (SOP) depends upon the pattern of the strabismus, and a summary of treatment strategies are listed in Table 8.3. Preoperative evaluation for inferior oblique overaction and superior oblique underaction is vital. Cardinal position of gaze measurements are also important to determine the pattern of strabismus and where the deviation is greatest. Most treatment strategies are based on where the deviation is greatest, and designing a surgical plan to correct the deviation in the primary position while reducing the incomitance. For example, a right unilateral superior oblique palsy with a hypertropia less than 18 to 20 PD, inferior oblique overaction, and minimal superior oblique underaction can be treated with a simple ipsilateral inferior oblique weakening procedure (e.g., inferior oblique recession with partial anteriorization). If the hypertropia in the primary position is greater than 20 PD, then an isolated inferior oblique recession will not be enough to correct the hypertropia. In this case one should add a contralateral inferior rectus recession, in addition to an ipsilateral inferior oblique recession. Late overcorrections after inferior rectus recessions have been known to occur, so be conservative with regards to recessing the contralateral inferior rectus muscle and consider using a nonabsorbable suture.

**TABLE 8.3.** Management of Superior Oblique Paresis

| Clinical manifestation | Procedure |
| --- | --- |
| *Unilateral Inferior Oblique Overaction* | |
| Hyperdeviation in primary position <18 PD | Ipsilateral inferior oblique weakening procedure (graded anteriorization) |
| Hyperdeviation in primary position >18 PD | Ipsilateral inferior oblique weakening with contralateral inferior rectus recession (if there is a significant hypertropia in down gaze) |
| *Bilateral SOP with Inferior Oblique Overaction* | |
| Hyperdeviation in primary position <8 PD | Bilateral inferior oblique graded anteriorization |
| *Masked Bilateral SOP* | |
| Hyperdeviation in primary position with asymmetric inferior oblique overaction. (See example figure 8.1 above) | Asymmetric bilateral inferior oblique graded anteriorization with greater anteriorization on the side of the hyperdeviation <br> plus <br> Inferior rectus recession on opposite side of the hypertropia |
| *Recovered Bilateral SOP (pure extorsion >8°)* | |
| Minimal hypertropia, <5 PD, small V-pattern and minimal inferior oblique overaction and superior oblique underaction | Bilateral Harada-Ito procedures. If a small hypertropia is present, do an asymmetric Harada-Ito by harnessing more of the superior oblique tendon on the side of the hypertropia |
| *Bilateral Severe SOP "Arrow" Pattern* | |
| Arrow pattern (>15 PD of esotropia in downgaze), >15° of extorsion in primary position increasing in down gaze. Reversing hypertropias in side gaze and superior oblique underaction. | Bilateral Harada-Ito procedures or bilateral superior oblique tendon tucks <br> plus <br> Bilateral medial rectus muscle inferior transposition 1/2 tendon width, or bilateral inferior rectus recessions |

## *Harada-Ito Procedure*

This procedure consists of selectively tightening the anterior one-quarter to one-third of the superior oblique tendon fibers. The Harada-Ito procedure acts to intort the eye, and slightly tightens the whole tendon, causing slight depression and abduction of the eye. The most important indication for a Harada-Ito procedure is to correct extorsion, but an ipsilateral Harada-Ito will also correct a small hypertropia (5 PD), and a bilateral Harada-Ito will improve 5 to 8 PD of a V pattern (Chapter 18). Patients with bilateral traumatic superior oblique paresis often have partial recovery and may be left with extorsion and esotropia in down gaze, without significant oblique dysfunction or a hypertropia in the primary position. These cases can be improved by bilateral Harada-Ito procedures (corrects the extorsion and some of the esotropia) with bilateral medial rectus recessions and infraplacement one-half of the tendon width (corrects the esotropia in down gaze).

## *Superior Oblique Tuck*

Tightening the entire width of the superior oblique tendon is termed superior oblique tuck and is of theoretical use for improving superior oblique function. A superior oblique tuck, however, results in minimal, if any, improvement of superior oblique function but produces a tight tendon and an iatrogenic Brown's syndrome.

Table 8.3 lists the treatment modalities for common presentations of superior oblique paresis.

## Sixth Nerve Palsy

The hallmark of a sixth nerve palsy is limited abduction. There is lack of abduction saccades, and force generation test shows deficient lateral rectus function (see Figure 8.2). Evaluation of lateral rectus function is imperative in making the appropriate procedural choice.

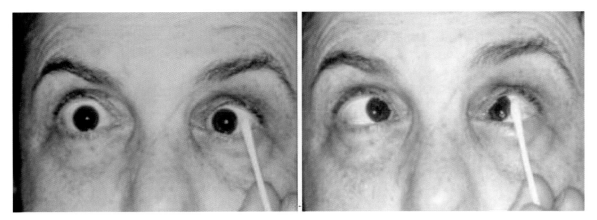

FIGURE 8.2. Traumatic left sixth nerve palsy with poor lateral rectus function as demonstrated by the force generation test. (*Left*): Topical anesthetic is instilled in the left eye and a cotton tip applicator is placed at the temporal limbus. (*Right*) Patient is asked to look to the left to activate the left lateral rectus muscle. The cotton tip applicator gently pushes against the eye to feel the abduction of the lateral rectus muscle. In this case, there is poor lateral rectus function, so the eye is held in adduction as the patient attempts to abduct.

### Initial Treatment

The initial treatment of an acquired sixth nerve palsy is observation for at least 6 months to allow for functional recovery. Botulinum toxin injection to the ipsilateral medial rectus muscle has been advocated to reduce secondary contracture of the ipsilateral medial rectus muscle and to reduce the need for subsequent strabismus surgery. Holmes et al, however, have found no significant improvement in outcomes after using botulinum toxin as an initial treatment.[2]

### Surgical Treatment

The surgical management of sixth nerve paresis is based on the amount of lateral rectus function present, and the size and pattern of the esotropia after the 6 months waiting period. See Table 8.4 for a summary of surgical

TABLE 8.4. Surgical Management of Sixth Nerve Paresis

| | | |
|---|---|---|
| A. | Good lateral rectus function | Bilateral medial rectus muscle recessions. If the esotropia is incomitant (and it usually is), then recess the contralateral medial rectus more than the ipsilateral medial rectus muscle. |
| B. | Fair lateral rectus function | Recess ipsilateral medial rectus muscle, resection of ipsilateral lateral rectus muscle, and small contralateral medial rectus recession with or without faden. |
| C. | Poor lateral rectus function | Ipsilateral medial rectus recession and Hummelsheim split tendon transfer with Foster modification |

strategies. An exception is the treatment of sixth nerve palsy associated with Möbius syndrome. Treat the large angle esotropia and apparent bilateral sixth nerve palsy by bilateral large medial rectus recessions (see Chapter 3 for Möbius syndrome).

## Good Lateral Rectus Function

In patients with good lateral rectus function (80% to 100% recovery) with an esotropia of 10 to 20 PD in the primary position and almost full ductions, consider performing bilateral medial rectus muscle recessions. If the esotropia is incomitant (and it usually is), then recess the contralateral medial rectus muscle more than the ipsilateral medial rectus muscle. For example, recess the contralateral medial rectus muscle 6.0 mm and the ipsilateral medial rectus muscle 3.0 mm for an esotropia of 20 PD in the primary position. The larger recession on the yoke muscle (i.e., contralateral medial rectus muscle) helps correct the incomitance. Some surgeons would add a faden to the contralateral medial rectus muscle.

## Fair Lateral Rectus Function

In patients with fair lateral rectus function (50% to 80%) with an esotropia >20 PD in the primary position and −2 limitation of abduction, consider recessing the ipsilateral medial rectus muscle and resecting the ipsilateral lateral rectus muscle. Also consider a contralateral medial rectus muscle recession (yoke to the paretic lateral rectus muscle) possibly with a faden. Weakening the contralateral medial rectus muscle helps to match the weak yoke function, thus improving lateral incomitance.

## Poor Lateral Rectus Function

If the lateral rectus function is poor (≤50% of normal), and abduction is −3 to −4, then an ipsilateral medial rectus muscle recession (adjustable suture) and a vertical muscle transposition procedure is indicated. There are two basic transposition procedures: the full-tendon transfer (Knapp procedure), and the split tendon transfer (Hummelsheim and Jensen procedures). The Knapp procedure is described for the treatment of double elevator palsy, but can be modified to treat sixth nerve palsies by transposing the superior and inferior rectus muscles laterally. A full tendon transfer disrupts major contributors to the anterior segment circulation and, therefore, carries a significant risk for anterior segment ischemia. Split tendon transfer procedures have the advantage of preserving half of the vertical rectus anterior ciliary vessels, reducing the incidence of postoperative anterior segment ischemia. A possible disadvantage of the split tendon transfer procedure is its reduced effectiveness. Split tendon procedures can produce strong abduction forces, if the muscle being transposed is fully mobilized, by splitting the muscle at least 14 mm posterior to the muscle insertion and by using the Foster modification (Chapter 16). Ipsilateral medial rectus recession and split tendon transfer of superior and inferior rectus muscles temporally (Hummelsheim procedure) with Foster modification is preferred by the author for patients with poor lateral rectus function.

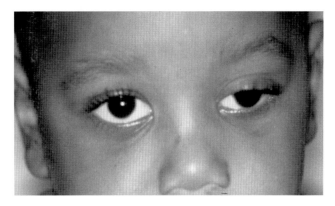

**FIGURE 8.3.** A left congenital third nerve palsy with ptosis, exotropia, and hypotropia (eye down and out).

## Third Nerve Palsy

There is a palsy of the superior, inferior and medial rectus muscles. The standard procedure for third nerve paresis with good to fair medial rectus muscle function is an ipsilateral lateral rectus recession and medial rectus resection (or plication). Add an ipsilateral superior oblique elongation procedure if a hypotropia is present. If the muscle function is poor a recess-resect procedure does not work for the long term. A vertical rectus transposition to the lateral rectus will also undercorrect the exotropia, as the transposed muscles are paralyzed. Superior oblique tendon transfer to medial rectus insertion has been described for exotropia with poor medial rectus function, however, limited depression and residual exotropia is common. Splitting the lateral rectus and transposing it to the nasal side of the superior and inferior rectus muscles, lateral rectus extirpation, or suturing the lateral rectus to the lateral orbital wall are other alternatives. These procedures leave the eye fixed in primary position. Ptosis is often present, and a silicone frontalis sling can be considered. If superior rectus muscle function is poor (no Bell's phenomenon), the patient is at risk for developing corneal exposure after the lid sling procedure. In these patients it is wise to undercorrect the ptosis to avoid exposure keratitis. Silicone material is preferred because it can be easily removed if corneal exposure occurs.

*Surgery for Complete Third Nerve Palsy (Exotropia and Hypotropia)*

- Recess lateral rectus muscle (12mm), resect medial rectus muscle (maximum), and do a superior oblique tenotomy or silicone tendon expander.
  Or
- Disinsert the lateral rectus muscle and attach it to the lateral orbital wall, and resect the medial rectus muscle.[3]
  Or
- Split the lateral rectus muscle for 14mm posterior to the insertion. Then transpose the upper half of the lateral rectus up and under the superior rectus muscle to reattach it 2mm posterior to the nasal pole of the superior rectus insertion. Transpose the lower half of the lateral rectus muscle under the inferior rectus muscle (between sclera and the IR muscle) and reattach it 2mm posterior to the nasal pole of the inferior rectus insertion. Resect the medial rectus muscle.

## Inferior Oblique Paresis

*Clinical Features*

- Limited elevation in adduction
- Marked superior oblique overaction
- Forced duction is negative
- A-pattern
- Positive head tilt test

Inferior oblique paresis is rare and can be confused with Brown's syndrome or primary superior oblique overaction (Figure 8.4). Unlike Brown's syndrome, there is superior oblique overaction, an A pattern, and forced ductions are negative. In contrast to primary superior oblique overaction, inferior oblique paresis is associated with a positive head tilt test, and the largest hyperdeviation occurs when the patient looks up and in. Inferior oblique paresis may be congenital or acquired. Congenital inferior oblique paresis is often unilateral, and associated with a large hypophoria in the primary position that can be fused. Patients with acquired inferior oblique paresis experience cyclo-vertical diplopia and require a neurological evaluation. The surgical treatment of unilateral inferior oblique paresis is an ipsilateral superior oblique weakening procedure such as the Wright's silicone tendon or split tendon elongation. A contralateral superior rectus recession is added if the hypotropia is 10 PD or more in the primary position (Table 8.5).

*Right Congenital Inferior Oblique Palsy*

| *Right gaze* | *Primary position* | *Left gaze* |
|---|---|---|
| LHT 5 PD | LHT 15 PD | LHT 25 PD |
| Head tilt right—LHT 5 PD | | Head tilt left—LHT 18 PD |

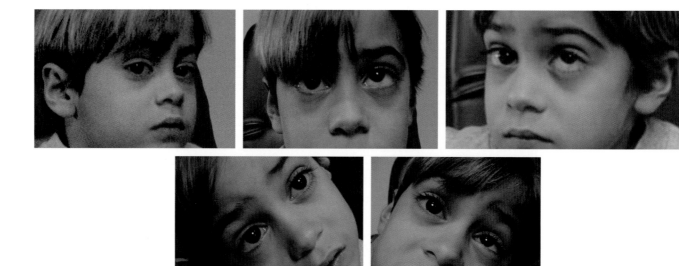

**FIGURE 8.4.** Composite photographs of a child with a right congenital inferior oblique palsy. There is a left hypertropia in the primary position that increases in left gaze and disappears in right gaze. Head tilt test shows the left hypertropia increases on tilt left. This patient had right superior oblique overaction +2.

**TABLE 8.5.** Surgery for Inferior Oblique Palsy

| Hypotropia <10 PD in primary position |
| --- |
| Ipsilateral Wright's superior oblique silicone tendon expander (5.0 mm to 6.0 mm) or superior oblique split tendon elongation |
| Hypotropia ≥10 PD in primary position |
| Ipsilateral Wright's superior oblique silicone tendon expander (6.0 mm to 7.0 mm) or superior oblique split tendon elongation with contralateral superior rectus recession |

# References

1. Helveston EM, et al. Surgical treatment of superior oblique palsy. Trans Am Ophthalmol Soc 1996;94:315–328; discussion 328–334.
2. Holmes JM, Leske DA, Christiansen SP. Initial treatment outcomes in chronic sixth nerve palsy. J AAPOS 2001;5:370–376.
3. Morad Y, Kowal L, Scott AB. Lateral rectus muscle disinsertion and reattachment to the lateral orbital wall. Br J Ophthalmol 2005;89:983–985.

# Section Two
## Surgical Techniques

# 9 Surgical Anatomy

An intimate knowledge of anatomy, including the extraocular muscles, periocular fascia, and orbit, is necessary to be an accomplished strabismus surgeon. This chapter reviews anatomical relations relevant to strabismus surgery.

## Muscle Measurements

The basic anatomic features of the extraocular muscles are summarized in Table 9.1. The four rectus muscles are essentially the same length (40 mm), although the amount of tendon varies, with the medial rectus having the shortest tendon length (4 mm), and the lateral rectus having the longest tendon length (8 mm). Of all of the extraocular muscles, the superior oblique has the shortest muscle length (32 mm) and the longest tendon length (26 mm), whereas the inferior oblique has only a 1 mm tendon. The distances in millimeters, in Table 9.1 and Figure 9.1, are for adults.

## Conjunctiva

It is often said that the conjunctiva is forgiving to the surgeon, but beware because poorly placed incisions can lead to functional and cosmetic problems. The plica, lateral canthus, and extraconal fat pad are important structures to avoid. Conjunctival incisions that extend into the plica are painful, causing unsightly scarring, and may cause a restrictive strabismus. Incisions that extend from the bulbar conjunctiva to the lateral canthus may cause symblepharon and restriction. In the inferior fornix, the extraconal fat pad starts approximately 10 mm posterior to the limbus, and can be identified as a soft bulge deep in the fornix. Fornix incisions should be placed anterior to this fat pad to avoid fat adherence and bleeding.

## Subconjunctival Fascia

### Muscle Pulley System: Muscle Sleeve

The extraocular muscles are held in place within the orbit by an intricate fascial network. This fascial network suspends the muscles as they approach the eye, and was termed "muscle sleeve" by the late Dr. Parks. The new term, popularized by Dr. Demer, is "muscle pulley" system.[1] In the anterior orbit, the pulley system holds the rectus muscles close to the orbital wall

**TABLE 9.1.** Extraocular Muscles

| MUSCLE | APPROXIMATE MUSCLE LENGTH (mm) | ORIGIN | ANATOMIC INSERTION (mm) | TENDON LENGTH (mm) | ARC OF CONTACT (mm) | ACTION FROM PRIMARY POSITION |
|---|---|---|---|---|---|---|
| Medial Rectus | 40 | Annulus of Zinn | 5.5 | 4 | 6 | Adduction |
| Lateral Rectus | 40 | Annulus of Zinn | 7.0 | 8 | 10 | Abduction |
| Superior Rectus | 40 | Annulus of Zinn | 8.0 | 6 | 6.5 | Elevation Intorsion Adduction |
| Inferior Rectus | 40 | Annulus of Zinn | 6.5 | 7 | 7 | Depression Extorsion Adduction |
| Superior Oblique | 32 | Orbit apex above annulus of Zinn | From temporal pole of superior rectus to within 6.5 mm of optic nerve | 26 / 1 | 12 / 15 | Intorsion Depression Abduction |
| Inferior Oblique | 37 | Lacrimal fossa | Macular area | | | Extorsion Elevation Abduction |

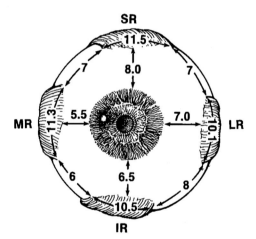

**FIGURE 9.1.** The rectus muscle insertions are horseshoe shaped, with the horse walking toward the limbus. The progressive increase of insertion distance from the limbus, with the medial rectus being the closest and the superior rectus being the farthest, is called the spiral of Tillaux. The surgeon should heed the posterior extension of the horseshoe insertion when passing a hook behind the muscle. The approximate tendon width, at the insertion, of each rectus muscle is 10 mm, and the average distance between rectus muscle insertions is 6 mm to 8 mm. Thus, even a half-tendon width transposition of any rectus muscle places it within a few millimeters of the adjacent rectus insertion. Because of the proximity of the muscles, it is possible to inadvertently hook the wrong rectus muscle during strabismus surgery.

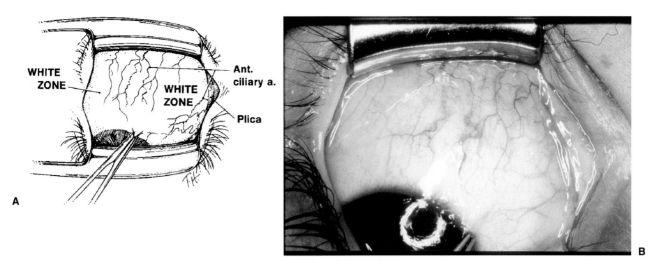

**FIGURE 9.2.** The drawing (**A**) and companion photograph (**B**) show the left inferior rectus muscle insertion and its anterior ciliary arteries as seen through the intact conjuntiva (surgeon's view). The rectus muscle insertions can usually be located before surgery by identifying their ciliary arteries, which are associated with a band of pink tissue. Anterior ciliary arteries lie deep below the conjunctival vessels and do not move if the conjunctiva is manipulated. Preoperative identification of rectus muscle insertions, and the white zone between the muscles, is important, as these landmarks guide the placement of the conjunctival incision and reduce the possibility of inadvertently hooking the wrong muscle. The white zone is the clear area between the rectus muscles. Sometimes it is difficult to positively identify the anterior ciliary arteries and the rectus muscles. The white zone, on the other hand, is a consistent landmark and can be identified in virtually all patients.

until the muscle exits the pulley to attach to the eyeball. Ectopic pulley location has been implicated as a cause of some types of incomitant strabismus.[2] Ectopic muscles have been a well documented cause of incomitant strabismus in patients with craniofacial synostosis. In these cases extorsion of the orbits is responsible for displacing the muscles.[3] The medial rectus muscles are displaced up and the lateral rectus muscles down, causing apparent inferior oblique overaction. The superior rectus muscles are displaced laterally and inferior rectus muscles nasally, producing a V pattern. These cases aside, ectopic pulleys, as a rule, are not a common cause of incomitant strabismus.

**FIGURE 9.3.** The relationship of the extraocular muscles to the intermuscular septum, Tenon's capsule, and orbital fat is depicted. Notice that this section is taken 12 mm posterior to the limbus, at the equator. The *Tenon's capsule* is the fascial layer that extends from the limbus to the optic nerve, and separates the orbital fat from the muscles and globe. The *intermuscular septum* is an extension of Tenon's capsule that connects the muscle. At the equator, intermuscular septum is sandwiched between Tenon's capsule on the outside and sclera on the inside. (See Figure 9.11 for sagittal cut through orbit.)

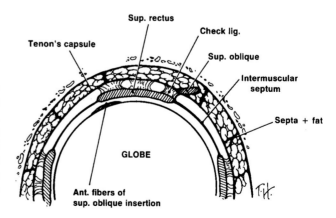

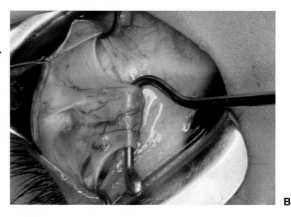

**FIGURE 9.4. (A)** The lateral rectus muscle is shown exiting the muscle sleeve (pulley). Check ligaments overlie the rectus muscles and connect the muscle to the overlying conjunctiva. The intermuscular septum is seen on each side of the muscle with wings spread, resembling the wings of a manta ray. Anterior Tenon's capsule extends anteriorly from the rectus muscles to the limbus. Anterior Tenon's capsule fuses with conjunctiva 1 mm from the limbus. **(B)** The Jameson hook is under the lateral rectus muscle and the Desmarres retractor is pulling the conjunctiva posteriorly.

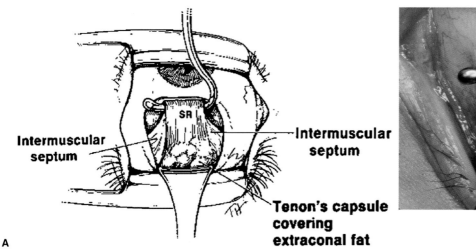

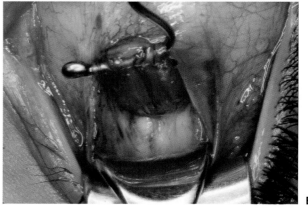

**FIGURE 9.5. (A)** The superior rectus muscle dissected free of check ligaments to expose the muscle as it penetrates Tenon's capsule approximately 12 mm posterior to the muscle insertion. In this area Tenon's capsule fuses with the intermuscular septum and forms the muscle sleeve. The muscle is attached to the muscle sleeve (pulley) by elastic check ligaments. Histologic studies of the pulley system have shown the presence of elastic tissue and smooth muscle.[1] If during strabismus surgery a rectus muscle is inadvertently severed and lost, it can retract through the muscle sleeve making retrieval difficult. **(B)** The superior rectus muscle with surrounding muscle sleeve. The muscle sleeve is the white shiny tissue between the Desmarres retractor and the superior rectus muscle. Extraconal fat is seen behind the muscle sleeve. The muscle sleeve with Tenon's capsule separates intraconal and extraconal orbit fat from the anterior muscle and sclera.

## Fat Adherence

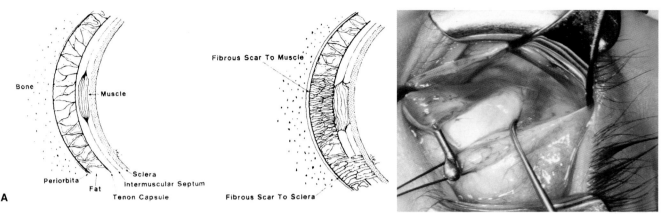

**FIGURE 9.6.** Violation of Tenon's capsule or muscle sleeve causes prolapse of orbital fat. Manipulated orbital fat can scar to the muscle or sclera, creating a restrictive band between periorbita (periosteum) and the muscle and/or sclera. This process is an important cause of restrictive strabismus and was termed fat adherence by Dr. Parks. Fat adherence is a common cause of restrictive strabismus after retinal detachment surgery but can be a complication of virtually any periocular surgery including strabismus surgery.[4] Once fat adherence occurs, the restriction of eye movement is extremely difficult to treat. Surgical removal of the adherence can improve ocular rotations but residual limitation is common. Prevent fat adherence by keeping the dissection of extraocular muscles close to the muscle belly to avoid violating Tenon's capsule and muscle sleeve.

## Individual Muscles

### Medial Rectus

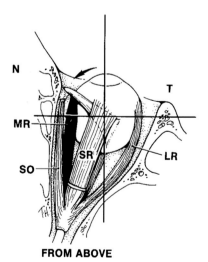

**FROM ABOVE**

**FIGURE 9.7.** The medial rectus muscle acts as a pure adductor. It has a "short" distinction, as it has the shortest arc of contact and is the shortest distance from the limbus. Because of the short arc of contact, the faden procedure is effective on the medial rectus muscle. Its insertion is closest to the limbus and is therefore easy to inadvertently excise from the globe during anterior segment procedures, such as pterygium removal, if one is not careful. The author has had patients with a lost medial rectus referred from experienced corneal surgeons.

The medial rectus muscle is the easiest muscle to lose and the hardest to find once lost, because is it the only extraocular muscle without fascial attachments to an oblique muscle. The muscle penetrates Tenon's capsule 12 mm posterior to its insertion and, if released, will retract posteriorly through the muscle sleeve making retrieval extremely difficult.

*Lateral Rectus*

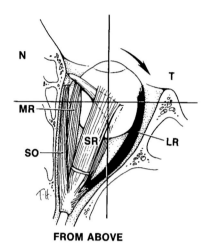

**FROM ABOVE**

FIGURE 9.8. The lateral rectus muscle acts as a pure abductor. Of the four rectus muscles, the lateral rectus has the longest arc of contact, making the faden operation on this muscle ineffective. The lateral rectus and inferior oblique muscles are joined by a ligament at the inferior oblique insertion. Because of this connecting ligament large hang back and adjustable suture recessions of the lateral rectus do not work well as the muscle will not retract posteriorly. A slipped or lost lateral rectus muscle will retract and then stop at the inferior oblique insertion. A lost lateral rectus muscle can usually be retrieved by tracing the inferior oblique muscle to its insertion.

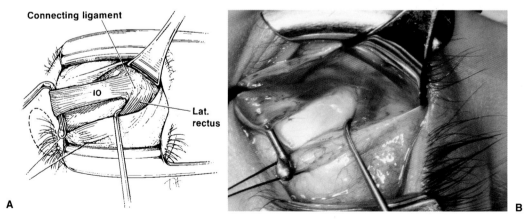

FIGURE 9.9. (A) The right inferior temporal quadrant with lateral rectus muscle and insertion site of the inferior oblique. Note the ligament connecting the inferior oblique and lateral rectus. (B) The right lateral rectus and inferior oblique are joined by a connecting ligament. A large Jameson hook is under the inferior oblique and is being pulled nasally while the lateral rectus is being retracted superiorly by a small Stevens hook and superonasally by a black silk traction suture, which is behind the lateral rectus insertion.

*Inferior Rectus*

FIGURE 9.10. The inferior rectus muscle is primarily a depressor but, depending on the eye's position, it can act as an adductor and extortor. These secondary actions occur because the muscle axis is 23° temporal to the visual axis when the eye is in the primary position. The inferior rectus muscle is a pure depressor only when the eye is abducted 23° from the primary position. Conversely, as the eye moves into adduction, the inferior rectus increasingly functions as an extortor and adductor.

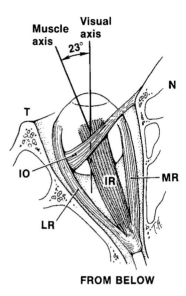

There are fascial connections between the inferior rectus, inferior oblique, and the lower eyelid retractors called the Lockwood's ligament (see Figure 9.12). This relationship is extremely important when performing surgery on the inferior rectus. The fascial connections between the inferior rectus and inferior oblique muscles are responsible for lower lid retraction after inferior rectus recession. Lower lid retraction can be minimized by removing the lower lid retractors. Connections between the inferior rectus and inferior oblique work to the surgeon's advantage when looking for a lost inferior rectus muscle. The inferior rectus muscle can often be retrieved by tracing the course of the inferior oblique muscle.

*Superior Rectus*

FIGURE 9.11. The superior rectus muscle is primarily an elevator, but also acts as an intortor and adductor in the primary position. The superior rectus is a pure elevator only when the eye is abducted 23°. As with the inferior rectus, there is a fascial attachment that connects the superior rectus with the upper eyelid elevators (see Figure 9.12). Eyelid retraction can occur after large superior rectus recessions, usually those over 5 mm. Careful removal of fascial connections can minimize this complication. The dissection should extend approximately 10 mm posterior to the muscle insertion. Special care must be taken during superior rectus surgery to avoid shearing off the anterior portion of the superior oblique insertion when removing intermuscular septum.

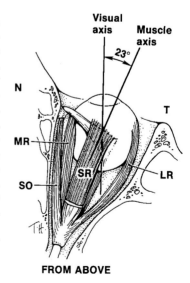

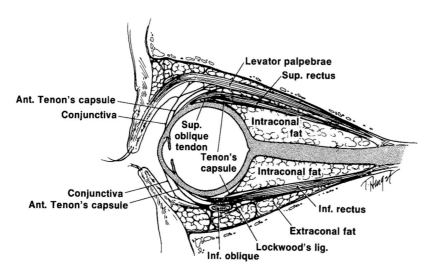

**FIGURE 9.12.** The drawing shows a sagittal view of extraocular muscles, orbital fat, and fascial attachments. Both vertical rectus muscles overlie the oblique muscles, with the inferior rectus sandwiched between the sclera above and the inferior oblique below, while the superior oblique is sandwiched between the superior rectus above and the sclera below.

### Inferior Oblique

The primary function of the inferior oblique is extorsion. It is also an abductor and elevator. The field of action of the inferior oblique is superior nasal (elevation in adduction), and this is the position of gaze in which the inferior oblique overaction is most noticeable. The inferior oblique muscle inserts directly over the macula, so inferior oblique surgery must be done with extreme caution to avoid scleral perforation and damage to the macula. The use of the Wright grooved hook (Titan Surgical, www.titansurgical.com, Los Angeles, CA), to suture the muscle insertion, helps protect against scleral perforation. The inferior temporal vortex vein is in close proximity to the inferior oblique muscle. The inferior oblique should be isolated on a hook under direct visualization to avoid disrupting the vortex vein. If the vortex vein is inadvertently damaged, cautery should not be used to stop the bleeding. The nerve innervating the inferior oblique enters the muscle approximately 15 mm nasal to the insertion.

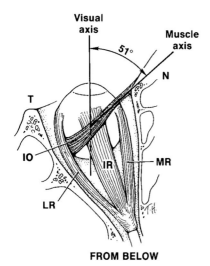

**FROM BELOW**

**FIGURE 9.13.** The function of the inferior oblique muscle is primarily as an extortor, but the muscle also acts as an abductor and elevator. In adduction, the inferior oblique functions more as an elevator and, in abduction, the muscle functions more as an extortor and abductor.

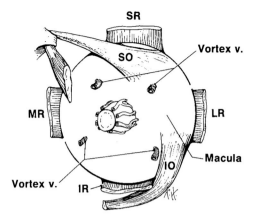

**FIGURE 9.14.** In this posterior-lateral view of the globe, notice the relationship of the inferior temporal vortex vein and the macula to the inferior oblique insertion.

## Superior Oblique

The superior oblique muscle is primarily an intortor, but also acts as an abductor and depressor in the primary position. There are two distinct parts of the superior oblique tendon: the cord portion and the fan portion. The round or cord portion of the superior oblique tendon passes through the trochlea and fans out just nasal to the superior rectus muscle. When the eye looks up and in, the cord portion elongates and passes through the trochlea. Restriction of superior oblique tendon movement is the most probable cause of Brown's syndrome. The fan portion of the tendon can be divided into the anterior one third and posterior two thirds. Anterior tendon fibers have intorsion function, while posterior tendon fibers are responsible for depression and abduction and, to a lesser degree, intorsion.

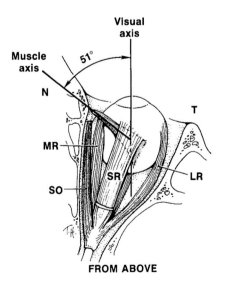

**FIGURE 9.15.** Top down drawing of the superior oblique muscle tendon complex. Note the posterior reflection of the tendon as it exits the trochlea.

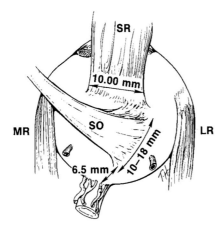

**FIGURE 9.16.** The insertion of the superior oblique is extremely broad. The anterior portion of this delicate fan-like insertion connects with the temporal insertion of the superior rectus muscle. These anterior fibers can be easily disrupted when isolating the superior rectus from the temporal side. The broad posterior insertion extends to within 6.5 mm of the optic nerve. During superior oblique surgery and exploration, care must be taken to avoid inadvertent damage to the optic nerve.

## Vascular Supply and Anterior Segment Ischemia

Disinserting a rectus muscle during strabismus surgery will interfere with the vascular supply to the anterior segment. Anterior segment ischemia is a well-known, albeit rare, complication of strabismus surgery. There is no formula for the number of rectus muscles that can be safely detached, but once a muscle with its anterior ciliary arteries has been detached, the vessels do not reestablish perfusion to the anterior segment. As a general

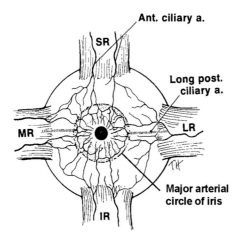

**FIGURE 9.17.** The anterior segment is fed by seven anterior ciliary arteries and two long posterior ciliary arteries, with approximately 50% perfusion from posterior ciliary arteries and 50% from anterior ciliary vessels. Two anterior ciliary arteries course through each rectus muscle, except for the lateral rectus muscle, which has only one artery. Anterior to the rectus muscle insertions, the anterior ciliary arteries branch to form the episcleral limbal plexus. This, in turn, connects to the major arterial circle of the iris, which is also fed by the two long posterior ciliary arteries. The long posterior ciliary arteries penetrate the globe close to the equator at 3 o'clock and 9 o'clock and course anteriorly to anastomose with the anterior circulation.

rule, do not detach more than two rectus muscles at one time, unless absolutely necessary. As the two vertical rectus muscles and the medial rectus muscle provide the major anterior ciliary blood supply to the anterior segment, try to preserve at least one of these muscles. It is important to note that anterior segment ischemia can occur years, and even decades, after the initial strabismus surgery. Factors that predispose to anterior segment ischemia include small vessel disease, hyperviscosity syndromes, and previous retinal detachment surgery with 360° scleral buckle.

## References

1. Demer JL, Miller JM, Poukens V, Vinters HV, Glasgow BJ. Evidence for fibromuscular pulleys of the recti extraocular muscles. Invest Ophthalmol Vis Sci 1995;36:1125–1136.
2. Oh SY, Clark RA, Velez F, Rosenbaum AL, Demer JL. Incomitant strabismus associated with instability of rectus pulleys. Invest Ophthalmol Vis Sci 2002;43:2169–2178.
3. Cheng H, et al. Dissociated eye movements in craniosynostosis: a hypothesis revived. Br J Ophthalmol 1993;77:563–568.
4. Wright KW. The fat adherence syndrome and strabismus after retina surgery. Ophthalmology 1986;93:411–415.

# 10 Basic Surgical Techniques (Do's and Don'ts)

## Setup and Exposure

Adequate surgical exposure is the key to any operation. Good exposure starts with proper positioning of the patient. The top of the head should be positioned at the very end of the surgical table, placing the neck in an extended position so the chin is higher than the forehead. Extending the neck lowers the superior orbital rim and eyebrow, improving exposure to the eye.

Surgical exposure is also facilitated by keeping the eye proptosed during surgery. Unknowingly, the eye may be pushed posteriorly while being rotated in an attempt to provide exposure. This reduces the exposure, forcing the surgeon to work in a "hole".

Holding the instruments away from the tips keeps the surgeon's and assistant's hands out of the surgical field. If the instruments are grasped close to the tips, the surgeon's view is blocked.

## Incision Options

There are four basic incisions for strabismus surgery: limbal, fornix, Swan, and combination fornix-Swan. Table 10.1 lists incision options for strabismus surgery.

### Limbal Incision

The limbal incision provides a large field of exposure and is probably the most popular worldwide. It consists of fornix wing incisions on one or both sides of the muscle and a limbal incision in front of the muscle (Figure 10.2). Patients who are more than 40 years of age have thin friable conjunctiva, and the limbal incision permits exposure without pulling or tearing the conjunctiva. Much has been said about the role of conjunctival recession in augmenting rectus muscle recession. Conjunctival recession increases the effect of the recession only if the conjunctiva is tight and is causing a restriction. In most pediatric strabismus cases, there is no conjunctival restriction and, therefore, conjunctival recession is rarely needed. In older patients with long-standing large deviations, the conjunctiva may be tight, in which case a conjunctival recession is indicated (e.g., tight contracted conjunctiva over the lateral rectus muscle in a large exotropia). Limbal incisions are essential if the conjunctiva is to be recessed due to tightness which is causing mechanical restriction of eye movement.

The limbal incision is preferred for horizontal rectus muscle surgery performed under topical anesthesia, as it provides good exposure without

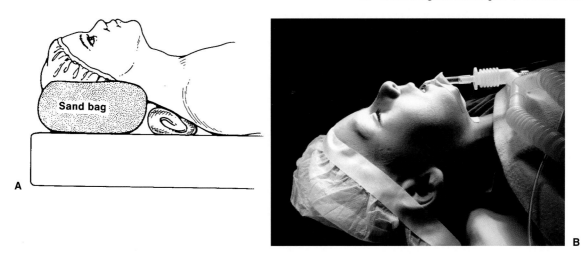

FIGURE 10.1. (A) A towel roll under the shoulders extends the neck, placing the chin higher than the forehead so the patient looks back toward the surgeon. Two sandbags on each side of the head are used to stabilize the head. Do not use a thick doughnut under the head, because it will elevate the head and reduce the neck extension. (B) Appropriate head position with the head gently stabilized with tape. Note that the breathing tube is flat so the surgical drapes will lie flat and out of the way.

TABLE 10.1. Incision Options

| Incision | Muscle surgery |
|---|---|
| Limbal | Rectus muscles at any age |
| Fornix | Rectus muscles <40 years of age |
|  | Oblique muscles at any age |
| Swan | Vertical rectus muscles at any age |
| Combination Fornix-Swan | Vertical rectus muscles at any age |
|  | Rectus muscles re-operation at any age |

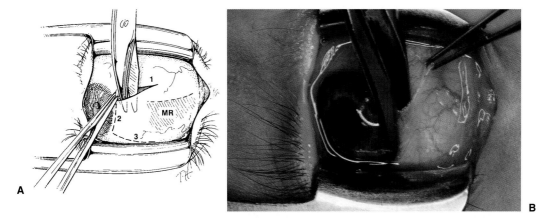

FIGURE 10.2. (A) The three steps of a limbal incision. First, make a radial wing incision in the fornix and extend it to the limbus. Second, perform a limbal peritomy right on the limbus in front of the muscle. Third, make the second radial wing incision above the muscle. The second wing incision is optional depending on the need for posterior exposure. (B) Photograph of step two, which is a limbal peritomy performed with the Westcott scissors.

pulling on the muscle. Disadvantages of the limbal incision include: possibility of a visible scar, dellen formation, more conjunctival scarring and discomfort than fornix surgery. See Chapter 11 for details regarding surgical technique.

### Fornix or Cul-de-Sac Incision

The fornix incision was developed by the late Dr. Marshall Parks. He summed up fornix surgery best by stating "fornix surgery is more difficult for the surgeon, but better for the patient." The incision is made between the rectus muscles in the fornix (Figure 10.3). Some call it peek-a-boo surgery because the incision is small and requires stretching the conjunctiva to gain exposure. The advantages of fornix surgery include patient comfort, the small incision scar that is hidden under the eyelid, the speed with which it can be performed, minimal scarring, and access to rectus and adjacent oblique muscles through a single incision in cases of A and V patterns. In re-operations, the fornix incision is excellent, as it gives the surgeon posterior exposure, facilitating muscle hooking and isolation without having to dissect the anterior conjunctiva off the sclera. The fornix incision is preferred for oblique muscle surgery, as it provides excellent exposure. The fornix incision is my incision of choice for horizontal rectus muscle surgery in patients less than 40 years of age, and for oblique muscle surgery in patients at any age. The disadvantages include inadvertent conjunctival tears and the relatively limited exposure for rectus muscles. See Chapter 11 for details regarding surgical technique.

### Swan Incision

Dr. Ken Swan from Portland, Oregon, developed this incision, which is made directly over the rectus muscle (Figure 10.4). The Swan incision provides excellent exposure and is very useful for re-operations, as it avoids manipulation of the scarred anterior conjunctiva. The problem with the Swan incision is its tendency to scar to the scleral insertion site if not closed well, thereby causing a cosmetic blemish. This can be a concern for

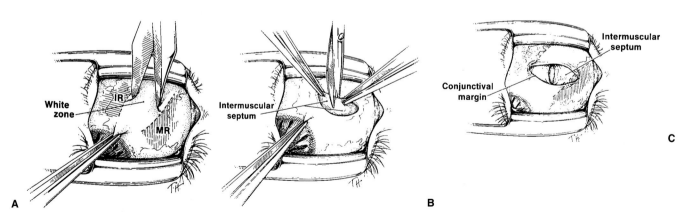

**FIGURE 10.3.** The fornix incision has two steps: (1) conjunctival incision and (2) intermuscular septum (anterior Tenon's capsule) incision. **(A)** An inferior nasal fornix conjunctival incision made between the inferior and medial rectus muscles with a blunt Westcott scissors. Note the incision is parallel to the lid speculum. **(B)** An incision through intermuscular septum (anterior Tenon's capsule). Note the incision is perpendicular to the conjunctival incision. **(C)** The fornix incision opening with the intermuscular septum incision perpendicular to the conjunctival incision.

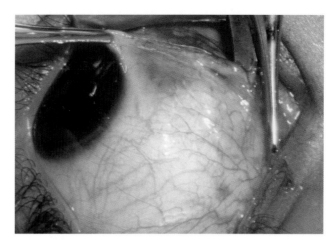

FIGURE 10.4. A Swan incision over the medial rectus muscle 2mm anterior to the plica.

horizontal rectus muscles, but not for the vertical rectus muscles, which are covered by the eyelid. Meticulous conjunctival closure is important when using the Swan incision. This photograph shows a Swan incision over the medial rectus muscle, used in a patient with previous strabismus surgery. Keep the incision anterior to the plica.

### Combination Fornix-Swan Incision

My preferred incision for vertical rectus muscles and re-operations with severe anterior scarring is a combination of fornix and Swan incisions. The incision starts at the fornix and goes down to the bare sclera; the muscle is then hooked. Once the muscle is hooked, the conjunctival incision is extended over the muscle insertion (Figure 10.5). This incision is particularly useful for surgery on patients who have had previous retinal detachment surgery with a scleral buckle, and for large recessions to gain posterior exposure. Careful conjunctival closure is important with this incision.

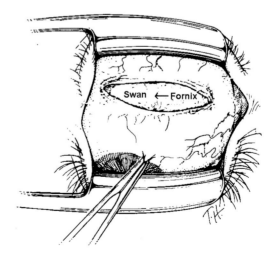

FIGURE 10.5. The combination fornix-Swan incision over the inferior rectus muscle.

## Hooking a Rectus Muscle

The surgeon uses a 2 × 3 Lester forceps to grasp the conjunctiva at the limbus, to retract the eye and expose the scleral quadrant between the muscles. The key to easy hooking of a rectus muscle is to gain access to bare sclera and the space beneath the intermuscular septum. Placing the hook on top of the intermuscular septum will keep the hook from passing under the muscle. One must stabilize the eye with the 2 × 3 Lester forceps. If the eye is free to move, hooking of the muscle will be more like bobbing for apples. Once bare sclera is identified, place the Stevens hook on the quadrant between the rectus muscles and orient the hook pointed down perpendicular to sclera (Figure 10.6). Pass the hook posterior and then rotate the hook underneath the border of the rectus muscle. Starting with the hook perpendicular to the sclera ensures that the tip of the muscle hook will remain in contact with the sclera and slide under the muscle. Once the muscle is hooked with the small hook, the 2 × 3 Lester forceps are released and a large Jameson hook is passed under the muscle to replace the Stevens hook (Figure 10.7). Make sure to keep the tip of the Jameson

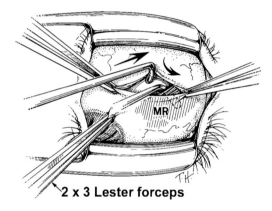

**2 x 3 Lester forceps**

**FIGURE 10.6.** The medial rectus being hooked with a small Stevens hook. Note that the hook is oriented perpendicular to sclera. Push the hook straight back behind the muscle insertion (approximately 7 mm), then rotate the hook up and under the muscle belly.

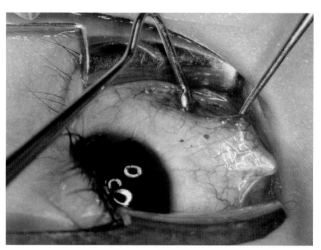

**FIGURE 10.7.** A small Stevens hook behind the medial rectus muscle pulling the muscle straight up off the sclera (to the ceiling) . A large Jameson hook is poised to be passed directly under the Stevens hook, parallel to the muscle insertion. After the Jameson hook is passed, the Stevens hook is removed.

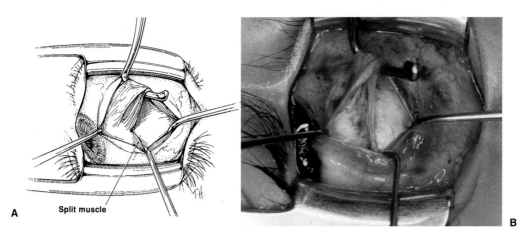

**A**  Split muscle

**B**

FIGURE 10.8. (A) Split Muscle: Drawing shows a positive pole test. The superior fibers of the left medial rectus have been split and the split muscle fibers are hooked by the Stevens hook. (B) The corresponding photograph shows a split medial rectus muscle. Note the main body of the medial rectus on the large Jameson hook, with the split fibers on the Stevens hook. If one is not careful, the split muscle could be misidentified as residual anterior Tenon's capsule or intermuscular septum.

hook against the sclera and parallel to the muscle insertion, to avoid splitting the muscle.

A rectus muscle may be inadvertently split during the process of hooking and isolating the muscle. If this is not identified, only part of the muscle will be operated on. The split muscle is best identified by the pole test (see Figure 10.8). The pole test is performed by placing two small Stevens hooks to expose the entire upper muscle pole (i.e., the end of the insertion). The hook closest to the cornea (i.e., the anterior hook) is kept perpendicular to, and directly on, sclera, then rotated anteriorly around the muscle pole. If the muscle is split, the Stevens hook will be trapped by the residual muscle fibers, limiting the advancement of the hook. To correct this situation, the residual muscle fibers are hooked with the small hook, elevated, and placed on the large hook with the main body of the muscle. Incorporate the split portion of the muscle with the rest of the muscle by placing the locking bite around the split and through the main portion of the muscle. There is really no harm done as long as the split muscle is identified and secured.

## Muscle Dissection

A rule of thumb regarding muscle dissection is to do as little "cleaning" as possible. When posterior muscle dissection is necessary (e.g., superior and inferior rectus recession, rectus resections, and some re-operations), removal of intermuscular septum and check ligaments should be done close to the muscle belly, to avoid penetration of posterior Tenon's capsule and manipulation of orbital fat. The dissection should be performed with blunt, curved Westcott scissors. Check ligaments are exposed using two small Stevens hooks or a Desmarres retractor to retract the anterior Tenon's capsule and conjunctiva up and off the muscle. Once on stretch, the check ligaments are removed close to the muscle belly, by both blunt spreading and sharp dissection. The intermuscular septum is removed in a similar manner, using the small Stevens hook to stretch the intermuscular septum and then removing the septum close to the muscle with sharp dissection.

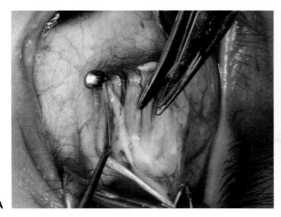 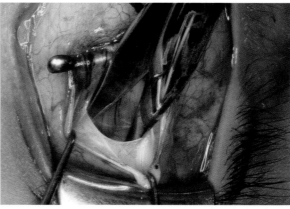

**FIGURE 10.9.** The dissection technique to clear check ligaments from the surface of the right superior rectus muscle includes the following: (**A**) Check ligaments are seen as the white tissue between the conjunctiva and the surface of the superior rectus muscle. Blunt dissection prevents bleeding and helps identify the dissection plane. (**B**) Blunt Westcott scissors are seen spreading through check ligaments with tips down on the surface of the muscle. Sharp cutting is used for residual fibers that are not removed by blunt dissection.

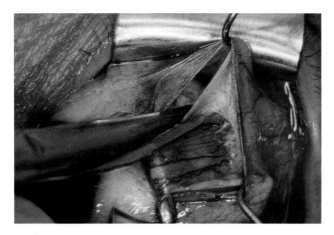

**FIGURE 10.10.** The intermuscular septum of the right lateral rectus is retracted off sclera with a Stevens hook. Blunt Westcott scissors are used to remove the intermuscular septum by cutting close to the muscle belly.

## Muscle Suturing Techniques

Successful strabismus surgery requires proper suturing of the muscle to prevent a slipped or lost muscle. The first step is the removal of the anterior Tenon's capsule from the tendon, to allow direct visualization of tendon fibers. If the anterior aspect of the muscle has too much residual Tenon's capsule, visualization of the true tendon is impossible, and sutures can be mistakenly placed through the anterior Tenon's without securing the muscle tendon. When the muscle is removed, it slips back posteriorly and the surgeon unknowingly secures the anterior Tenon's capsule to the sclera. This produces a slipped muscle, causing postoperative overcorrection for recessions, and undercorrections for resections.

Another important step is suturing the muscle properly, so the muscle fibers are well secured. Muscles are made up of longitudinal contractile fibers. Partial thickness suture bites secure only the superficial fibers, leaving the rest of the fibers free to slip posteriorly after the muscle is removed (Figure 10.11). Securing deep fibers is an essential part of stra-

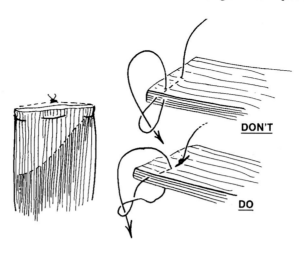

FIGURE 10.11. Drawing to the left shows a muscle that slipped partially because the deep muscle fibers were not secured. The top right drawing shows what not to do, as there is a thin partial thickness pass through the muscle, and no twist to the suture lock. Often, the surgeon thinks the muscle is secured, but the deep fibers are not locked, and they slip posteriorly, producing an undesirable postoperative result. Pass the needle perpendicular to the surface of the muscle throughout the entire needle pass for a full thickness locking bite. Do not slant the needle anteriorly until it has passed through the full thickness of the tendon. Bottom right drawing demonstrates how to make a large full thickness locking bite with a suture twist.

bismus surgery. Also secure the locking bites with a twist lock. The posterior retraction of muscle fibers, that occurs immediately after surgery because of faulty suturing of the muscle fibers, is termed slipped muscle. Ludwig and Chow described late posterior slippage of the muscle, what they call stretched scar. This represents a remodeling of the scar adhesion of the muscle to sclera. Release of the absorbable suture before the muscle fully adheres to the sclera, at usually 4 to 8 weeks after surgery, is a major contributing factor.[1] Late overcorrection commonly occurs after inferior rectus recession at 4 to 8 weeks after surgery.[2] The incidence of late overcorrection after inferior rectus recession for thyroid related strabismus is extremely high, and has been reported to be approximately 50% using Vicryl absorbable suture.[3] Some strabismus surgeons recommend reducing the recession when operating on thyroid patients. Others have advocated always doing bilateral inferior rectus recessions for thyroid strabismus, so if the muscle slips, both slip, and there would not be an induced hypertropia. This author now uses nonabsorbable sutures for securing the inferior rectus muscle in thyroid cases, to reduce the incidence of late overcorrection (see later in this chapter).

To improve outcomes many strabismus surgeons, including myself, have changed the suturing techniques for securing rectus muscles. We now suture all rectus muscles with three point fixation (Figure 10.12). Place a

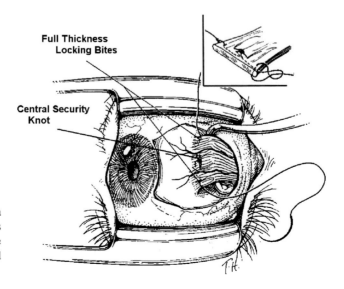

FIGURE 10.12. Three point fixation with a central security knot and large full thickness locking bites at each edge of the muscle. Use three point suture fixation for both recessions and resections.

"large" 3 mm central security knot full thickness, in the center of the muscle, tied in a square knot. Then two "large" 3 mm full thickness locking bites are placed at each edge of the muscle. It also helps to place a full twist in the lock knot to prevent the lock from loosening. This technique secures almost all of the 10 mm wide rectus muscle.

The suture material I use has also recently changed. I now use 5-0 Vicryl suture for standard rectus muscle surgery instead of a 6-0 Vicryl. In cases prone to stretched scar, such as thyroid cases, inferior rectus surgery in general, or advancement of a previously slipped or lost muscle, the author now uses nonabsorbable 5-0 Mersilene suture. When using a nonabsorbable suture, direct the scleral pass posteriorly so the knot ends up posterior to the new insertion. This helps to cover the knot and prevent late knot erosion through the conjunctiva (see Scleral Needle Pass later in this chapter).

### Wright Grooved Hook

Another modification for securing the muscle is the use of the Wright grooved hook (manufactured by Titan Surgical, www.titansurgical.com). The author developed this grooved hook (patent pending) that provides a space between the muscle and sclera to allow for safe suturing of full thickness muscle (Figure 10.13). The groove guides the needle pass protecting the eye from inadvertent needle puncture, while providing consistent suture placement with respect to the scleral insertion. Standard strabismus hooks (Green and Jameson) require the surgeon to lift the muscle upwards, off the sclera to expose the muscle for suturing. The Wright hook facilitates exposure as the muscle is pulled flat into the center of the surgical field, rather than up off the sclera as with standard hooks (Figure 10.14). The Wright hook is especially helpful for tight muscles.

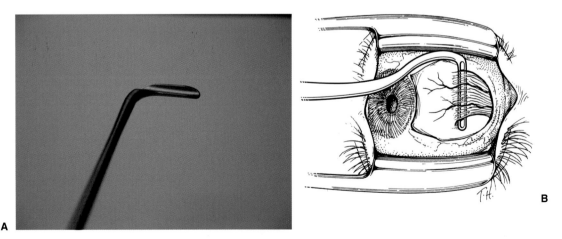

**FIGURE 10.13. (A)** The Wright grooved hook. Note that the groove is tilted toward the handle. This allows for suturing of the muscle close to the scleral insertion. **(B)** The Wright grooved hook under a rectus muscle. You suture directly over the groove.

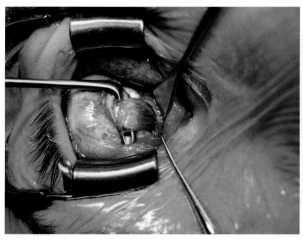
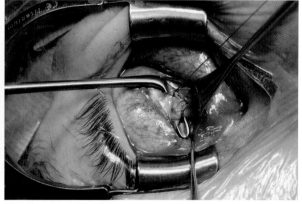

FIGURE 10.14. (A) The Wright grooved hook behind a tight medial rectus muscle that had been previously recessed. Note that the hook exposes the tight muscle as the surgeon pulls the muscle into the surgical field, rather than up off the sclera as with standard hooks (e.g., Jameson or Green). The groove allows for safe suture pass through the muscle for the full thickness central security knot, and locking bites at each edge of the muscle. (B) The Wright grooved hook and three point suture fixation; Central security knot and locking bites at the muscle edge. The grooved hook provides space under the muscle to facilitate full thickness suture passes, and to protect the sclera from inadvertent needle perforation.

## Scleral Needle Pass

The scleral pass is an important aspect of strabismus surgery, because inadvertent perforation can lead to retinal detachment and, rarely, endophthalmitis. Unlike other ophthalmic surgery, scleral passes in strabismus surgery are usually performed behind a rectus muscle insertion in the thinnest part of the sclera (approximately 0.3 mm thick). Because of the thin sclera, superficial passes with a spatula needle (i.e., side cutting) are mandatory to avoid scleral perforation (Figure 10.15).

When approaching the sclera with a needle, keep the needle tip up. The needle tip should be directed up until the curve of the needle touches the sclera. Then rotate the needle holder slightly to direct the needle tip into the sclera. A curved needle holder allows the needle to be splayed perpen-

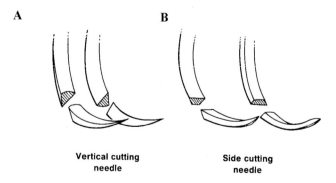

FIGURE 10.15. A vertical cutting needle (A) cuts vertically down (*left*) or up (*right*) and is inappropriate for scleral passes. A side cutting or spatula needle (B) is flat on the top and bottom surfaces, minimizing the likelihood of scleral perforation or cutting of a scleral tunnel.

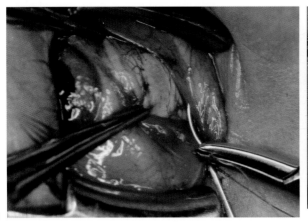
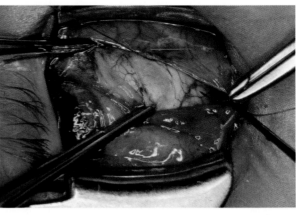

**FIGURE 10.16.** **(A)** The correct method for posterior exposure and scleral pass. Do retract conjunctiva, intermuscular septum, and rectus muscle out of the way with a small Stevens hook held flat on the sclera. A curved needed holder is used, and the needle approaches the eye tip up with the curve away from the sclera. **(B)** The incorrect method for posterior exposure and scleral pass. Do not lift the conjunctiva off the sclera, because this creates a hole that makes the scleral pass difficult. The straight needle holder improperly directs the needle tip straight down on approach to the sclera, increasing the risk of scleral perforation if the patient suddenly bucks or if a forceps slips.

dicular to the outside curve, which facilitates positioning the needle flat on the sclera. The scleral pass should be so superficial that the needle produces a bump in the sclera during the pass; pass like a mole, not like a gopher. To gain posterior scleral exposure, retract the conjunctiva and intermuscular septum posteriorly, keeping the Stevens hook tight against the sclera (do not lift up). Lifting the conjunctiva off sclera produces an obstruction and forces the surgeon to work in a narrow hole (Figure 10.16).

The usual scleral pass is directed anteriorly toward the cornea as seen in Figure 10.17. This technique puts the suture knot anterior to the muscle and is appropriate for absorbable sutures. Nonabsorbable suture knots, however, have a propensity for eroding through the conjunctiva over a period of several months. To reduce late erosion, aim the needle passes posteriorly so the knot resides behind the new muscle insertion (Figure 10.18).

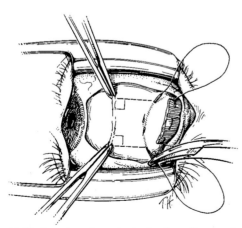

**FIGURE 10.17.** Drawing of standard scleral needle pass aimed anteriorly toward the cornea. This is the technique used for most recessions using absorbable sutures.

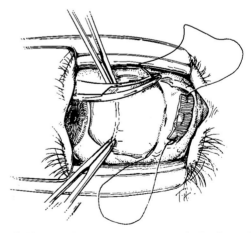

**FIGURE 10.18.** Drawing demonstrates posteriorly directed needle passes, to keep the knot posterior and to bury the knot under the muscle. This technique is used to keep the nonabsorbable suture knot from eroding through the conjunctiva.

## Pearls for Muscle Recession

### Central Muscle Sag

If a rectus muscle is not widely splayed, there will be redundant muscle and central sag causing a larger recession than intended. Prevent central sag by adequately separating the muscle poles and by securing the center of the muscle with a central security knot. Central sag can be corrected with the same suture that holds the muscle, but do not cut the sutures and needles off the knot (Figure 10.19).

### Loose Pole Suture

Occasionally, while tying the muscle in place, a suture will slip, causing a muscle pole to slip posterior to the desired location. This can be rectified by passing one end of the knotted double arm suture just anterior to the scleral insertion line.

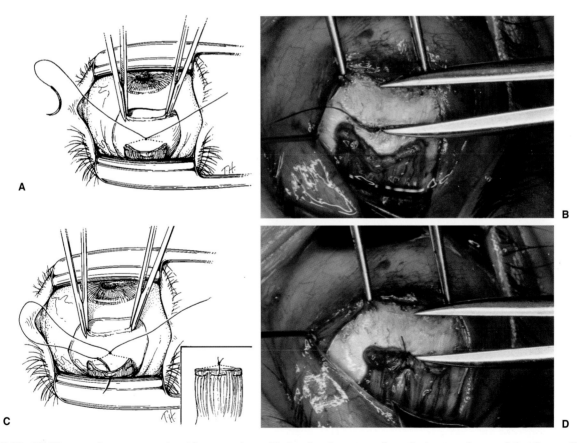

FIGURE 10.19. (A) The superior rectus mucle with a central sag. Notice that the sutures from the knot are long and that the needle was left on one of the ends of the suture. (B) A corresponding photograph shows that superior rectus muscle with 3 mm of central sag. The calipers are marking the intended recession, but the central portion of the muscle is posterior to this mark. (C) While the needle is still attached to the scleral knot, pass one end of the suture through the central aspect of the muscle belly, behind the original suture. Pull up on the suture to advance the central aspect of the muscle. Tie the two ends of the sutures together to hold the muscle in place. The inset shows the end result, with the central suture supporting the middle of the muscle. (D) The photograph shows the superior rectus muscle after the central muscle sag has been corrected. Calipers document that the appropriate recession has been made.

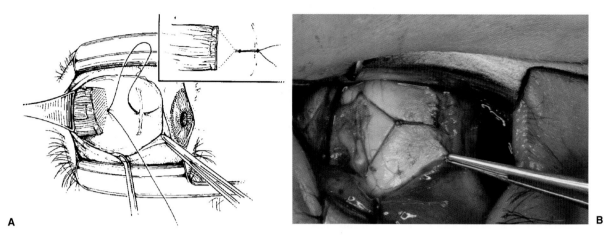

**FIGURE 10.20.** (**A**) The diagram shows slipped inferior pole of a right medial rectus muscle. The suture from the knotted double arm suture is passed at the scleral insertion line. Pulling up on this suture tightens the loose suture and advances the muscle pole. The inset shows the original knot advanced toward the insertion, thus advancing the muscle pole. (**B**) The photograph shows the suture configuration after suture advancement to take up suture slack.

## Forced Duction Testing

### Rectus Muscles

Forced ductions of the rectus muscles should always be performed if there is evidence of limited ductions or incomitance. If the eye is inadvertently pushed posteriorly into the orbit during the forced ductions maneuver, the rectus muscles will slacken, causing the ductions to feel normal, even in the presence of a tight rectus muscle. Positive forced ductions, that do not improve when the eye is intentionally retropulsed, suggest the presence of a nonrectus muscle restriction, such as periocular adhesion (e.g., fat adherence or fibrotic band), or a tight oblique muscle such as a tight superior oblique muscle in Brown's syndrome.

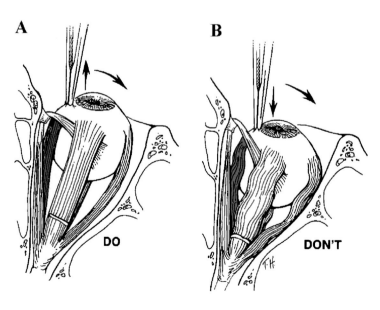

**FIGURE 10.21.** (**A**) Drawing demonstrates the technique for rectus muscle forced ductions by grasping the conjunctiva with 2 × 3 Lester forceps at the limbus, where the conjunctiva is adherent to the sclera. First, proptose the eye, and then pull the eye away from the muscle being tested, thus placing the rectus muscle on stretch. The maneuver allows identification of even mildly tight or restricted muscles. The medial rectus muscle (shaded muscle) in this drawing is tight. (**B**) The incorrect technique to test rectus muscle restriction is shown in drawing B. Note that the eye is retropulsed causing iatrogenic slackening of the rectus muscles resulting in a normal forced duction test even though the medial rectus is tight.

**FIGURE 10.22.** An anterior fibrotic adhesion from the nasal bone to globe. Note that forced ductions are positive whether the eye is proptosed (**A**) or retropulsed (**B**). This indicates a nonrectus muscle restriction; a leash from the bone to the globe.

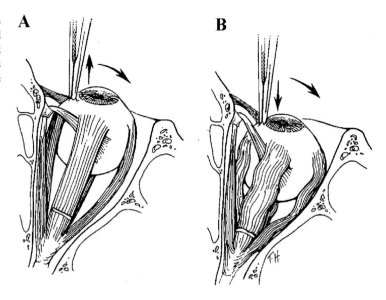

### Oblique Muscles

The tension or tightness of an oblique muscle can be tested by forced ductions using the exaggerated traction test developed by Dr. David Guyton.[4] The superior oblique is used as an example, but the same principles can be applied to the inferior oblique.

### Superior Oblique Tendon

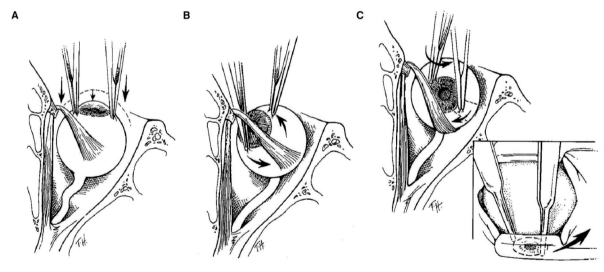

**FIGURE 10.23.** Place the superior oblique tendon on stretch by grasping the eye at 3 o'clock and 9 o'clock with deep fixation forceps (e.g., 0.5 Castroviejo forceps), and push the eye straight back in the orbit (**A**). Retropulsing the eye stretches the oblique muscles and slackens the rectus muscles. While retropulsed, the eye is adducted and then extorted until the tension from the superior oblique is felt (**B**). While maintaining a retropulsed and extorted position, the eye is swept from the medial canthus, superotemporally toward the lateral canthus, with the cornea following the arc of the superior orbital rim (**C**). During this maneuver, a firm bump can be felt as the superior oblique tendon slides over the top of the globe. The eye will almost stop, then roll over the tendon with a characteristic bump. As seen from the surgeon's view, the eye moves smoothly along the upper orbital rim toward the lateral canthus until the superior oblique tendon slips over the top of the globe (**C inset**).

Maintain slight extorsion tension throughout the sweep, in order to feel the tendon bump. If this maneuver is performed after a complete superior oblique tenotomy, the eye can be smoothly swept up and out, all the way to the lateral canthus without a tendon bump. This is a very specific and sensitive test for confirming that the entire superior oblique tendon has been cut.

## *Inferior Oblique Muscle*

The inferior oblique muscle is placed on stretch by retropulsion, and the eye is adducted and intorted. The eye is then swept from the medial canthus inferotemporally toward the lateral canthus. A bump can be felt during this maneuver as the inferior oblique slides over the inferior aspect of the globe. The bump from the inferior oblique is smoother and more subtle than that of the superior oblique tendon.

## References

1. Ludwig IH, Chow AY. Scar remodeling after strabismus surgery. J AAPOS 2000;4:326–333.
2. Wright KW. Late overcorrection after inferior rectus recession. Ophthalmology 1996;103:1503–1507.
3. Hudson HL, Feldon SE. Late overcorrection of hypotropia in Graves ophthalmopathy. Predictive factors. Ophthalmology 1992;99:356–360.
4. Guyton DL. Exaggerated traction test for the oblique muscles. Ophthalmology 1981;88:1035–1040.

# 11  Rectus Muscle Recession

Below is a detailed description of the rectus muscle recession procedure. Two conjunctival approaches are presented: Fornix and Limbal.

## Fornix Surgery

The fornix incision is somewhat difficult to learn but, when mastered, provides an excellent approach to the extraocular muscles. Unlike the limbal approach, the fornix incision is tucked away under the lid, and patients are very comfortable postoperatively. Because the limbal conjunctiva is intact, dellen formation is eliminated and cosmetic results are excellent. The fornix approach facilitates reoperation, especially when the first operation was a limbal surgery, because the fornix incision is behind the muscle insertion. This avoids an anterior conjunctival scar and permits direct access to the muscle. Dr. Marshall M. Parks developed the very elegant fornix approach described in this chapter.

The strategy for obtaining proper exposure with the fornix approach is to rotate the muscle into the incision while stretching the incision towards the muscle insertion. Once the surgeon and assistant establish their team approach, the fornix approach provides excellent exposure. Fornix incisions should usually be avoided in patients older than 40 years of age because the conjunctiva is thin and friable. (See Chapter 10 for more on conjunctival incisions).

The fornix approach gives access to at least two muscles with a single incision. An inferior nasal incision gains access to the inferior and medial rectus. An inferior temporal incision provides access to the inferior rectus, lateral rectus, and the inferior oblique. A superior temporal incision allows access to the superior rectus, lateral rectus and the superior oblique tendon. A superior nasal incision provides access to the medial rectus, superior rectus and the nasal aspect of the superior oblique tendon. For horizontal rectus surgery, it is advisable to place the incision in the inferior fornix.

Regardless of the incision, posterior dissection or "cleaning" of the intermuscular septum and check ligaments is not indicated and does not enhance the recession. Recessions of the superior and inferior rectus muscles require some posterior dissection of fascial attachments to prevent secondary lid changes (see Vertical Rectus Muscle Recession at the end of this chapter).

### Surgical Technique

The fornix approach is demonstrated for a left medial rectus recession (surgeon's view).

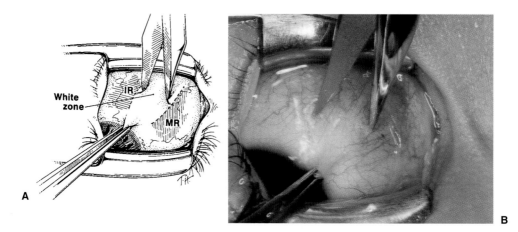

**FIGURE 11.1.** (**A**) A 2 × 3 Lester forceps rotates the eye up and out to expose the inferior nasal quadrant and stabilize the eye. The incision is made by cutting straight down through the conjunctiva in the white zone between the inferior rectus and medial rectus muscles, approximately 8 mm posterior to the limbus. Extend the conjunctival incision from the inferior rectus muscle to within 1 mm to 2 mm of plica. (**B**) The location and alignment of the initial incision. Notice that the incision line is parallel to the lid speculum and just anterior to the orbital fat pad. Avoid cutting into the orbital fat and plica.

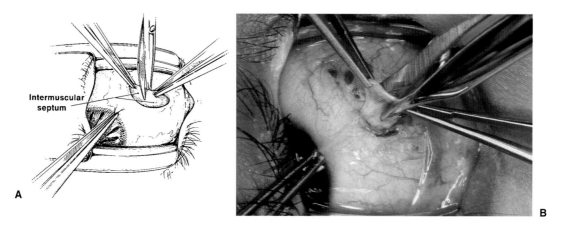

**FIGURE 11.2.** (**A**) With the eye drawn up and out, two 0.3 Castroviejo forceps pick up the intermuscular septum to form a tent, parallel to the conjunctival incision. Blunt Westcott scissors incise the intermuscular septum by cutting down over the tent, keeping both tips firmly against the sclera. This technique produces an incision in the intermuscular septum, perpendicular to the conjunctival opening. By keeping the scissors tips firmly on sclera, a single snip will cut through all layers of intermuscular septum and gain immediate access to bare sclera. Only the blunt Westcott scissors are used for cutting through intermuscular septum on to sclera. (**B**) The blunt Westcott scissors making an incision through the intermuscular septum.

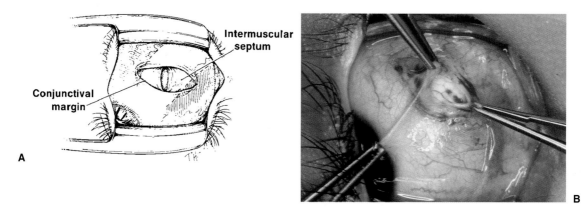

**FIGURE 11.3.** (**A**) The locations of the horizontal conjunctival incision, and the vertical incision through the intermuscular septum. It is important to cut down through full-thickness intermuscular septum to expose bare sclera. (**B**) The fornix incision, exposing bare sclera. The two forceps are grasping intermuscular septum.

**FIGURE 11.4.** With 2 × 3 Lester forceps stabilizing the eye in elevation and abduction, the medial rectus is hooked with a small Stevens hook. Place the Stevens hook directly perpendicular to sclera and pass the hook posteriorly and then superiorly, rotating the hook underneath the inferior border of the medial rectus muscle (*arrows*). Starting with the hook perpendicular to the sclera ensures that the tip of the muscle hook will remain in contact with the sclera and slide under the muscle.

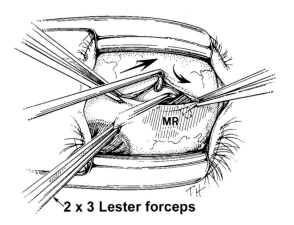

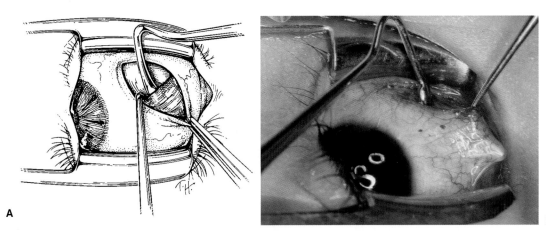

A                                        B

**FIGURE 11.5.** **(A)** Once the muscle is hooked with the small hook, the 2 × 3 Lester forceps are released and a large Jameson hook is passed under the muscle to replace the Stevens hook. Make sure to keep the tip of the Jameson hook against the sclera and perpendicular to the muscle fibers to avoid splitting muscle. **(B)** A small Stevens hook behind the medial rectus, pulling the muscle straight up off the sclera. A large Jameson hook is poised to be passed directly under the Stevens hook, parallel to the muscle insertion. After the Jameson hook is passed, the Stevens hook is removed.

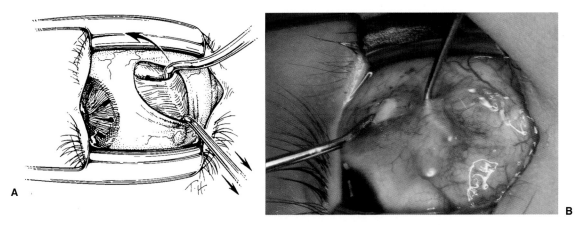

A                                        B

**FIGURE 11.6.** **(A)** Once the muscle is hooked, the conjunctival incision is reflected over the tip of the Jameson hook to expose the muscle. Place the small hook at the nasal end of the conjunctival incision and, keeping the hook flat on the surface of the muscle, pull the conjunctiva over the end of the Jameson hook. This is a bimanual technique, with the Jameson hook rotating inferiorly and temporally towards the incision while the small Stevens hook simultaneously pulls the conjunctiva superiorly over the tip of the Jameson hook (*arrow*). **(B)** A small Stevens hook underneath the conjunctiva, slowly slipping the conjunctiva toward the bulb tip of the Jameson hook. The Jameson hook simultaneously rotates inferiorly and temporally so that the bulb tip rotates toward the incision. Keep the tip of the Jameson hook up to prevent the muscle from slipping off the end of the hook.

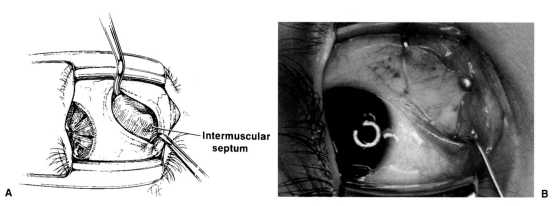

**FIGURE 11.7.** **(A)** The small hook folds the conjunctiva over the bulb tip of the Jameson hook. Notice the perpendicular position of the tip of the small hook, which is now facing the end of the Jameson hook. The tissue over the end of the Jameson hook is superonasal intermuscular septum. **(B)** The conjunctiva reflected over the end of the Jameson hook. The Jameson hook is directed tip up and rotated inferiorly into the area of the initial incision. The white tissue emanating over the bulb tip of the Jameson hook is superonasal intermuscular septum.

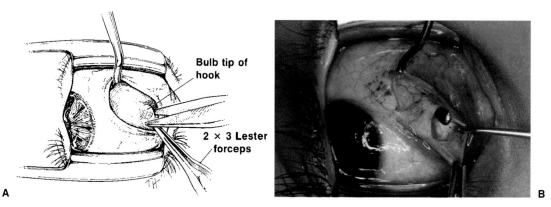

**FIGURE 11.8.** **(A)** The 2 × 3 Lester forceps are used to grasp the intermuscular septum (not the conjunctiva) at the end of the Jameson hook, and the small Stevens hook is removed from the conjunctiva. A hole in the intermuscular septum, between the bulb of the Jameson hook and the tip of the 2 × 3 Lester forceps, is cut with the Westcott scissors. The remnant of intermuscular septum is swept over the bulb of the Jameson hook to bare the end of the hook. **(B)** The bared bulb end of the Jameson hook. Notice that the 2 × 3 Lester forceps continue to pull intermuscular septum superiorly, opening the hole in intermuscular septum. A small Stevens hook is placed within the hole onto sclera to maintain the opening in intermuscular septum.

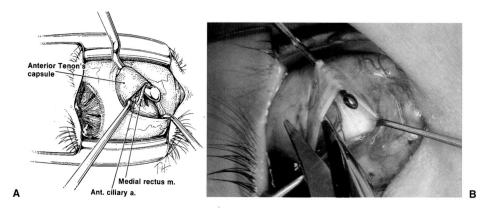

**FIGURE 11.9.** **(A)** A second Stevens hook is inserted into the hole in intermuscular septum, down to bare sclera. With the tip of this hook firmly on the sclera, it is swept anteriorly around the superior pole of the medial rectus muscle insertion. This maneuver of sweeping around the superior muscle pole is called the "pole test." If the muscle is inadvertently split, superior fibers of the medial rectus will snag the small hook as it sweeps anteriorly. A restricted pole test indicates residual muscle is not on the hook and a split tendon is present (see Figure 10.8). The Stevens hook pulls the anterior Tenon's capsule so it can be excised with the Westcott scissors. **(B)** The Westcott scissors removing anterior Tenon's capsule from the medial rectus tendon. The pole of the medial rectus tendon is identified by the presence of an anterior ciliary artery emanating off the tendon insertion. The blade of the Westcott scissors is slid between anterior Tenon's capsule and medial rectus tendon to excise anterior Tenon's capsule. Be careful not to inadvertently cut conjunctiva or tendon. The Stevens hooks are rotated together in front of the rectus muscle tendon to expose and excise the entire width of anterior Tenon's capsule. This maneuver cleans the muscle insertion so sutures will be passed through true tendon rather than the anterior Tenon's capsule, which could cause a slipped muscle.

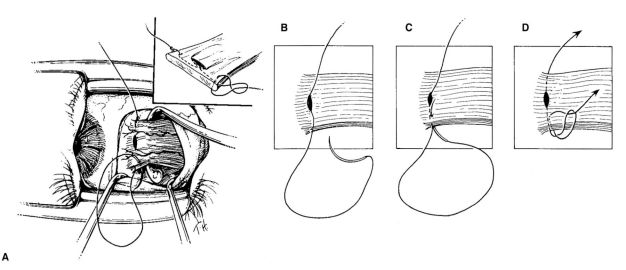

FIGURE 11.10. **(A)** Once the muscle is cleared of anterior Tenon's capsule it is secured with a single 5-0 or 6-0 Vicryl double arm suture with spatula needles (S-29 or S-24). The author's preference is now 5-0 Vicryl to provide stronger and longer lasting attachment. Two Stevens hooks are used to expose each muscle pole for the needle pass. It is important to keep the eye proptosed during all maneuvers and to rotate the muscle into the incision for better exposure. The muscle is sutured with three-point fixation; a central security square knot and a full thickness twist knot at each edge of the muscle. The drawing shows the full thickness locking bite being passed at the superior pole of the muscle. Note that passing full thickness is difficult because of the crowded area of folded muscle. We now use the Wright grooved hook for suturing the muscle, as it provides excellent muscle exposure and protects the sclera from inadvertent needle perforation (see Figures 11.11 and 11.12). Standard suturing technique: To minimize the incidence of slipped muscle or stretched scar, suture all rectus muscles with three-point fixation and 5-0 Vicryl suture. **(B)** Shows the first step being a deep, almost full thickness, central security knot. With the grooved hook the central bite can be deep and full thickness as the hook protects the sclera. **(C)** After the central security knot continue with a partial thickness pass starting from the center to periphery then a full thickness "large" 3 mm locking bite at the edge of the muscle. **(D)** Place a locking twist knot to secure the muscle edge. Use a full twist to make sure the knot will hold. The partial thickness pass from center to periphery is then repeated for the other side of the muscle.

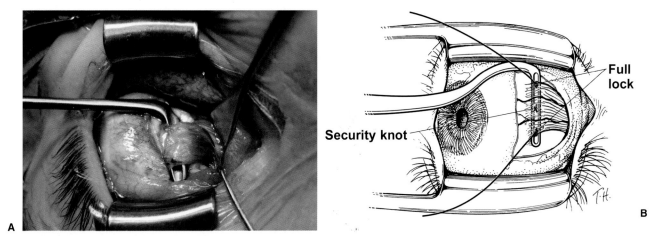

FIGURE 11.11. **(A)** A demonstration of the technique for securing the muscle using the Wright grooved hook. This case is a reoperation on a tight medial rectus muscle that had been previously recessed. Note the grooved hook behind the muscle, pulling the muscle temporally into the surgical field for optimum exposure. The groove is 12.5 mm long so it overlies the conjunctiva obviating the need for retraction hooks. The muscle is ready for suturing over the groove. Suturing over the groove hook allows for safe full thickness needle passes as the sclera is protected. **(B)** The Wright grooved hook with three-point suture fixation: Central security knot and locking bites at each edge of the muscle. The groove guides suture placement for reproducible location of suture bites 2 mm posterior to the scleral insertion. Use the same suturing weave to secure the muscle as described in Figure 11.10.

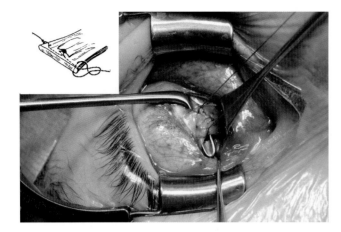

**FIGURE 11.12.** The three-point suture fixation (5-0 Vicryl) with a central security knot and full thickness locking bites at each end of the muscle insertion. The inset drawing shows the full thickness locking bites and central security knot.

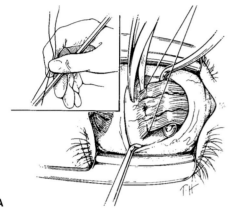

A

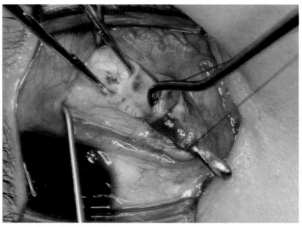

B

**FIGURE 11.13.** **(A)** Once the muscle is secured with Vicryl suture, the sutures are pulled tight and directed superiorly just over the Jameson hook. As the muscle is disinserted with the Westcott scissors, keep the sutures taut between two fingers to prevent sag and inadvertent cutting of the suture (*inset*). The muscle should be removed, flush on sclera. Do not leave a muscle stump, because a stump may be seen through the conjunctiva, causing a cosmetic blemish. **(B)** After the inferior half of the muscle is removed, place 0.5 Castroviejo locking forceps at the inferior end of the scleral insertion line. The forceps are best applied by sinking the single tooth posteriorly into the sclera and closing the other two teeth over the single tooth engaged in the sclera. The locking forceps stabilize and control the eye while the second half of the muscle is removed.

After the muscle is completely disinserted, place a second 0.5 Castroviejo locking forceps at the superior end of the scleral insertion line. It is important to identify and secure both ends of the scleral insertion line with locking forceps. Locking forceps identify the insertion line, control the eye position, and hold the conjunctival incision open to provide scleral exposure.

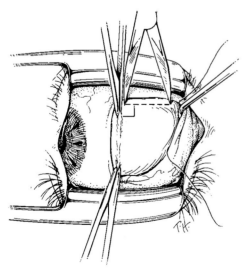

**FIGURE 11.14.** Two locking forceps are in place at each end of the scleral insertion line. Calipers are used to mark off the recession. Keep the calipers 90° to the scleral insertion line. When marking for muscle reattachment, make sure that the marks for the two muscle poles are separated by a full tendon width (approximately 10mm). Spreading the muscle will prevent central sag (see Chapter 10 for the treatment of central sag).

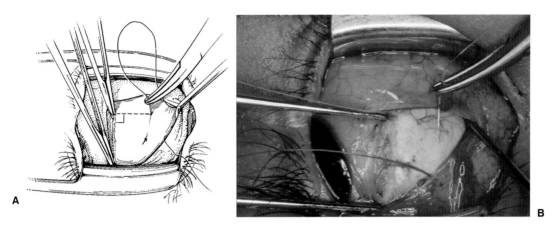

FIGURE 11.15. (A) The eye is rotated superiorly to expose the inferior aspect of the sclera. A small Stevens hook is used to retract conjunctiva posteriorly, and the S-29 spatulated needle is presented to the sclera. Keep the tip up as the needle approaches the sclera to avoid inadvertent perforation should the patient move. The S-29 needle can be passed slightly at an angle and does not have to be absolutely flush to the sclera. The key to this maneuver is to rotate the eye superiorly for the inferior needle pass, while retracting conjunctiva posteriorly with the small Stevens hook flat on the sclera. Do not lift up with the Stevens hook, as this elevates the conjunctiva and creates a hole, making the scleral pass extremely difficult. Keep the eye proptosed to improve access to the sclera. (B) The eye rotated superiorly, the globe proptosed, and a small Stevens hook retracting conjunctiva posteriorly, flat against sclera. Notice the shallow depth of the scleral needle pass. This is important, as the sclera is extremely thin behind the insertion (approximately 0.3 mm).

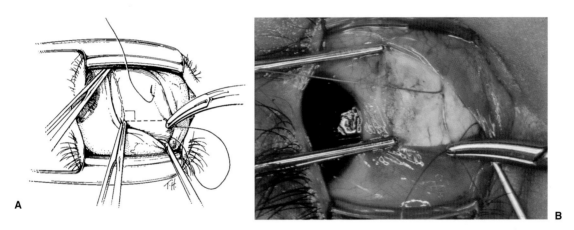

FIGURE 11.16. (A) Superior scleral passes are performed with the eye rotated inferiorly to expose superior sclera. The passes are directed parallel to the scleral insertion line, so the needles exit close together in a modified crossed-swords configuration. For large recessions through the fornix, it is best to remove each needle as it is passed to avoid the needle getting caught behind a fold of conjunctiva. (B) The superior scleral pass with the tip of the needle exiting close to the first suture.

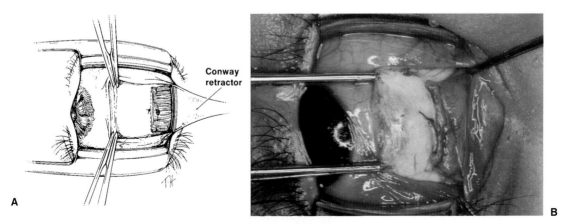

FIGURE 11.17. (A) The sutures are pulled to advance the muscle, and the medial rectus muscle is tied in place with three overhand knots. A small Stevens hook or a Conway retractor retracts the conjunctiva to provide posterior exposure. The muscle should be splayed out widely to avoid central sag. (B) The muscle widely splayed in place after recession with two Stevens hooks retracting the conjunctiva.

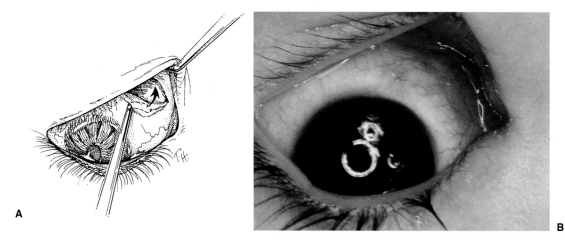

**FIGURE 11.18.** **(A)** The locking forceps and lid speculum have been removed from the eye. The conjunctiva is replaced by elevating the lower lid with a Jameson hook while a small Stevens hook is used to push or "snowplow" the anterior folds of conjunctiva posteriorly. The author now routinely closes the Tenon's intermuscular septum and conjunctiva with 6-0 plain gut to avoid the possibility of late Tenon's prolapse. **(B)** The conjunctival incision closed in the fornix. Suture the cut edges of the intermuscular septum together first, then close the conjunctiva separately. This provides a two-layered closure and prevents prolapse of redundant intermuscular septum.

## Limbal Surgery

Of all the conjunctival techniques, the limbal incision provides the broadest exposure of the rectus muscles and is the simplest to learn. The limbal incision works extremely well in patients who are more than 40 years of age and who often have friable conjunctiva that easily tears when stretched, as in fornix surgery. In older patients, the limbal approach is the surgery of choice, usually performed with a double wing incision. (See Chapter 10 for more on conjunctival incisions.)

*Surgical Technique*

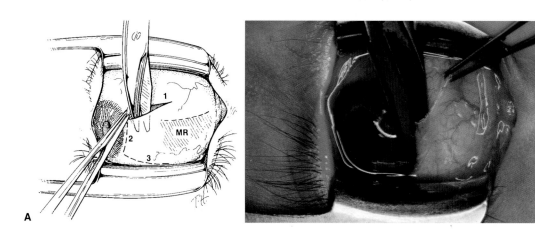

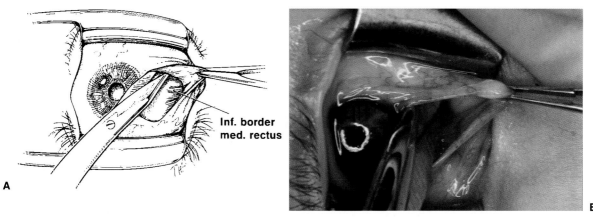

**FIGURE 11.20. (A)** The conjunctiva and Tenon's capsule are grasped in the area of the inferior nasal fornix, and the tissues are pulled straight up to expose the inferior nasal quadrant. The blunt Westcott scissors are closed, advanced along bare sclera into the inferior nasal quadrant, and then spread to open a small hole under intermuscular septum. **(B)** The inferior nasal quadrant with Westcott scissors exposing bare sclera.

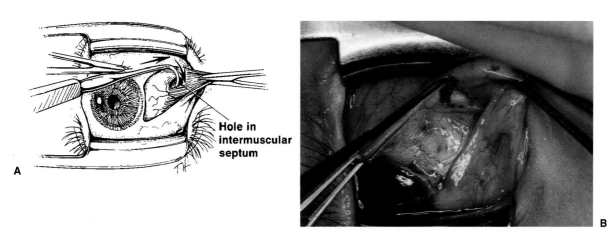

**FIGURE 11.21. (A)** The 2 × 3 Lester forceps are placed at the inferior limbus to stabilize and abduct the eye, while the inferior nasal conjunctiva and Tenon's capsule are grasped with 0.3 Castroviejo forceps and retracted to expose the inferior nasal sclera. The inferior pole of the medial rectus is identified by the anterior ciliary artery. Under direct visualization of the inferior pole of the medial rectus muscle, a small Stevens hook is placed perpendicular to sclera and passed behind the medial rectus muscle. The key in hooking a muscle is to start with the hook perpendicular to sclera, push posteriorly, and turn the corner behind the muscle. **(B)** The inferior nasal quadrant and inferior pole of the medial rectus muscle, along with one of its anterior ciliary arteries. Note how the Stevens hook is placed perpendicular to sclera, just posterior to the anterior ciliary artery and muscle insertion. It is important to have the tip of the small hook on bare sclera in order to get under the rectus muscle.

**FIGURE 11.19. (A)** Limbal approach, double wing incision for left medial rectus recession is demonstrated.

1. First, an inferior radial incision is performed. It is often necessary to make a second incision through Tenon's capsule to establish a scleral plane.
   *Option:* After step 1 and the scleral plane has been achieved, immediately hook the rectus muscle insertion. Then, using the hooked muscle to control eye position, continue with steps 2 and 3. This option allows control of eye position without using a forceps that can tear anterior conjunctiva.
2. Second, Westcott scissors are used to undermine the anterior Tenon's capsule and conjunctiva. Once the conjunctiva is freed, a limbal peritomy close to the sclera is performed over 4 clock hours.
3. Finally, a second radial incision is performed parallel to the first incision below.

**(B)** Limbal peritomy close to the sclera performed with blunt Westcott scissors.

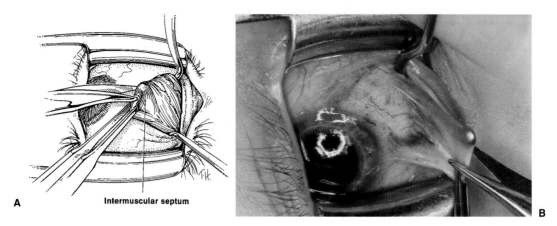

**FIGURE 11.22.** **(A)** The medial rectus muscle has been hooked within the Jameson hook, and the superior nasal intermuscular septum is folded over the tip of the Jameson hook. Intermuscular septum is incised by grasping below the tip of the muscle hook with a 2 × 3 Lester forceps and cutting between the forceps and the tip of the muscle hook. **(B)** Photograph shows 2 × 3 Lester forceps grasping intermuscular septum, which is coming off the top of the Jameson hook. Westcott scissors are used to open the intermuscular septum, bearing the muscle hook and exposing bare sclera.

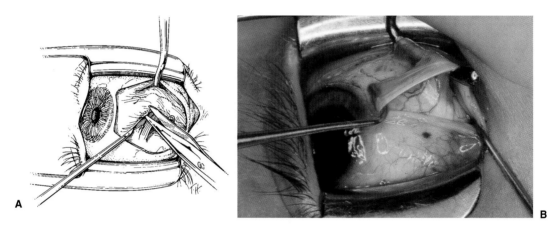

**FIGURE 11.23.** **(A)** The Westcott scissors are used to remove anterior Tenon's capsule. Tenon's capsule is placed on stretch as the small Stevens hook pulls the anterior Tenon's capsule away from the muscle insertion. The anterior Tenon's capsule should be cut close to the muscle. **(B)** Anterior Tenon's capsule swept anterior to the muscle insertion with the Stevens hook. Notice that all the fibers of the superior pole of the medial rectus are incorporated within the Jameson hook and there are no residual muscle fibers superior to the hook. Anterior ciliary arteries can be seen coming off the superior pole of the muscle.

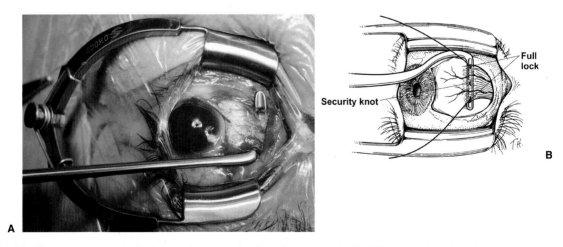

**FIGURE 11.24.** **(A)** Once the muscle is cleared of the anterior Tenon's capsule, the Wright grooved hook replaces the Jameson hook for suturing of the muscle. In this photograph, the Wright grooved hook is behind the muscle. **(B)** Drawing shows suturing of the muscle with a central security knot and full thickness locking bites at each edge of the muscle. Once the muscle is secured the muscle is disinserted from the sclera as described for fornix surgery above (see Figure 11.13).

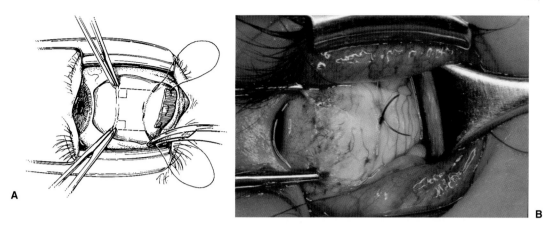

FIGURE 11.25. (A) Intrascleral needle passes are now placed superficially in a direction parallel to the insertion line. The scleral entrance point is the point to which the muscle will advance. Make sure to place the initial bites square to the insertion lines, so that the muscle will be appropriately splayed. The initial scleral bites should be separated by the width of the muscle insertion (approximately 10 mm). If the needle passes are placed too close together, the muscle will be bunched in the center and retract posteriorly (see Chapter 10 for management of central sag). (B) The photograph shows the crossed-swords technique. Notice that the needle passes are parallel with the insertion line and that the needles exit in a crossed-swords configuration. In performing very large recessions, it may be advisable to remove the first needle before making the second scleral pass, because the needle left within the sclera can get caught in the posterior conjunctiva and Tenon's capsule.

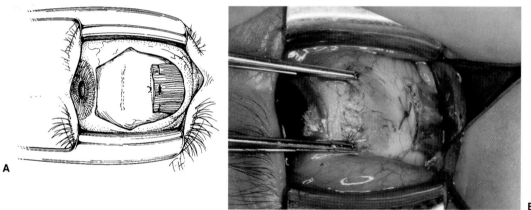

FIGURE 11.26. (A) The muscle is tied in place with three overhand knots, widely splayed out to approximately the same width as the scleral insertion line. The suture tags should be 2 mm long. (B) The photograph shows the muscle in place, splayed out widely, with no central sag. If the muscle is splayed out to approximately the same width as the original insertion, there will be no central sag.

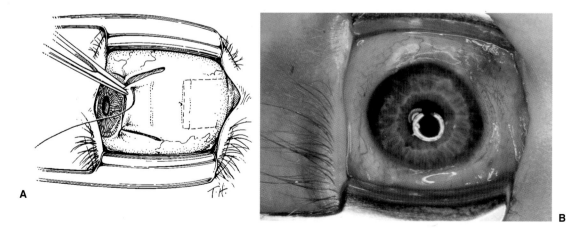

FIGURE 11.27. (A) Conjunctival closure is done using 6-0 plain gut suture. No conjunctival recession was performed in this patient, because the conjunctiva was not contracted or scarred. (B) Photograph at the end of the case, with conjunctival wings sutured. Antibiotic steroid combination ointment is placed in the eye and no patch is used.

*Dellen Formation*

An important albeit infrequent complication of the limbal incision is dellen formation. A dellen is corneal thinning at the limbus that stains to fluorescein. Dellens occur next to a conjunctival elevation, usually a lump of conjunctiva caused by a tight suture. The cause is a disruption of the normally uniform tear film. The first line of treatment is to pressure patch the eye or use artificial tears. If the dellen persists remove the conjunctival lump.

## Hang-Back Technique

As a rule this author tries to avoid the hang-back technique because of its inherent instability. The hang-back technique tends to produce overcorrection for small recessions (<5 mm), as there always is central sag. Central sag is avoided in the fixed-suture technique because the muscle poles are splayed out widely and anchored to sclera. For large recessions, hang-back recessions tend to creep forward, reducing the intended recession. The most a normal rectus muscle can be recessed with a hang-back suture is approximately 6 mm, unless the muscle is tight and contracted. Another problem is the potential for late slippage or stretched scar because the muscle is not secured to sclera. Except in specific circumstances as detailed below, it is far better to suture the muscle directly to sclera at the intended recession location.

The hang-back technique can be extremely useful for operating on strabismus associated with retinal detachment surgery. Often, the 360° silicone band is in the way of scleral passes. The hang-back technique allows fixation of the sutures anterior to the scleral buckle, with the muscle slung back over the buckle. Hang-back sutures may be nonabsorbable to facilitate retrieval of the muscle if a reoperation is necessary. The hang-back technique is important for cases predisposed to scleral perforation, such as high myopia and other cases where the sclera is thin. Hang-back is also useful for cases in which it is difficult, or impossible, to make a posterior scleral pass and the muscle is tight so it will retract posteriorly.

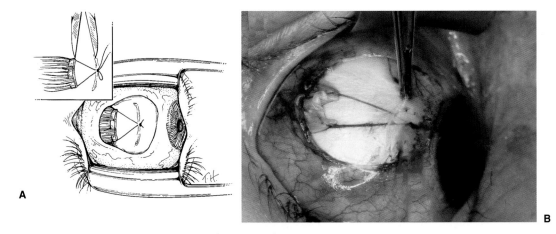

**A**    **B**

**FIGURE 11.28. (A)** The muscle is secured in the standard fashion by double-arm sutures. The two needles are passed through the center of the scleral insertion (approximately 3 mm apart) with the needles pointing toward each other to form a "V" with the apex oriented toward the cornea. Drawing of the muscle in the hang-back position suspended from the scleral insertion site. The inset shows the muscle slung posteriorly with the bow-tie at the scleral insertion. A caliper is used to confirm the recession by measuring posteriorly. The knot is tied with three overhand knots, and excess sutures are removed. **(B)** Photograph of a rectus muscle on a hang-back suture. Note the central sag.

# Vertical Rectus Muscle Recession

## Superior Rectus Muscle

The superior rectus muscle has fascial connections to the superior oblique muscle below, and the levator muscle above. Recession of the superior rectus muscle can result in upper lid retraction, as the posteriorly placed superior rectus muscle will pull the upper lid back. A posterior dissection of eyelid attachments to the superior rectus muscle is important to avoid lid retraction after a superior rectus recession. Dissect close to the superior rectus muscle to avoid penetrating muscle sleeve and Tenon's capsule. Violation of Tenon's capsule can result in fat adherence to the muscle or globe, causing postoperative restriction.

## Inferior Rectus Muscle

There are fascial attachments of the inferior rectus muscle to the lower eyelid. The inferior rectus muscle, inferior oblique muscle, and the lower lid have a unique anatomical relationship, as they are interconnected by the lower lid retractors (capsulo-palpebral system). This is a continuous musculo-tendonous tissue that arises from the inferior rectus muscle posterior to the inferior oblique, courses anteriorly to envelope the inferior oblique muscle, then continues anteriorly to insert into the tarsal plate. Lockwood's ligament is the enveloping tissue around the inferior oblique that unites the tarsus to the inferior rectus muscle. Recession of the inferior rectus muscle will result in lower lid retraction, as the inferior rectus muscle pulls the lower lid retractors posteriorly via Lockwood's ligament. The standard approach to minimize lid retraction is to perform a posterior dissection for 10 mm to 15 mm along the inferior surface of the inferior rectus muscle to remove the attachments to the lower lid. This extensive dissection causes scarring and even fat adherence, and usually does not prevent postoperative lower eye lid retraction. It is important to dissect close to the inferior rectus muscle to avoid penetrating Tenon's capsule and exposing orbital fat. Instead of the extensive dissection, we now do a small inferior rectus dissection for 5 mm to 6 mm but routinely disinsert the lower lid retractors. Removal of lower lid retractors has significantly improved the problem of lower lid retraction.

## Lower Lid Retractor Disinsertion

We usually disinsert the lower lid retractors when performing inferior rectus recessions of 5 mm or more. This can be done rather simply. First place a 4-0 silk traction suture 2 mm below the lash line in the middle of the lid. Pass the suture deep enough to secure the superficial layers of the tarsal plate. Then place a large Desmarres retractor behind the suture to evert the lid to show the tarsal conjunctiva and the inferior border of the tarsal plate. The lower lid retractors insert at the inferior border of the tarsal plate. Lower lid retractors are removed from the tarsus by using the cut/coagulation mode of a Colorado needle. Pass the Colorado needle 1 mm to 2 mm below the inferior border of the tarsus to burn through the conjunctiva and underlying lid retractors. Remove the retractors for most of the 10 mm length of the tarsal plate. Do not go too deep or you can burn the underlying skin. For inferior rectus recessions greater than 5 mm consider placing a reverse Frost suture to hold the lower lid up, to keep the lid retractors separated from the tarsus. The Frost suture should be left in place for approximately 24 hours.

# 12 Topical Anesthesia Strabismus Surgery

Topical anesthesia strabismus surgery reduces the systemic risk, as well as the postoperative nausea and vomiting associated with general anesthesia. It also eliminates the risk of globe perforation, optic nerve damage, and myotoxicity that is associated with retrobulbar injection. Topical anesthesia can be especially useful in senior citizens who have medical issues that make general anesthesia dangerous.

The author reserves topical anesthesia for cooperative adult patients and only for virgin rectus muscle recessions, including bilateral surgery and vertical or horizontal rectus muscle surgery. Others (probably braver and more skilled surgeons) have used topical anesthesia for resections. Topical anesthesia works well for rectus muscle recessions in patients with thyroid related strabismus.

## Principles for Avoiding Pain

Pain during strabismus surgery originates from two main sources: the conjunctiva and the extraocular muscles. Manipulation of the Tenon's capsule and sclera, however, does not result in pain. Grasping the scleral insertion with locking forceps and scleral needle passes can be performed safely without discomfort.

The conjunctiva can be anesthetized with topical anesthesia using tetracaine and lidocaine gel. We use multiple doses of both topical tetracaine and lidocaine gel prior to surgery. The extraocular muscles provide a more difficult hurdle, as we cannot anesthetize the muscles without a retrobulbar injection. Pain from the extraocular muscles does not arise from pain receptors, as cutting the muscle or passing a needle through the muscle is not painful. Muscle pain comes from stretch receptors and is elicited by pulling on the muscle. Even gentle pulling on a rectus muscle will cause significant pain. This is a gut wrenching deep visceral pain, which must be avoided. Once the patient experiences pain from muscle pull, confidence will be lost, making the rest of the surgery miserable for both the surgeon and patient alike.

Standard strabismus surgery is based on pulling on the muscle to gain muscle exposure, so special techniques are required for topical anesthesia to minimize muscle pull. First, avoid the fornix approach, as this approach requires significant pulling on the muscle. Use a limbal or Swan incision to gain wide and easy access to the muscle insertion. The author prefers the limbal incision for the horizontal recti and the Swan incision for vertical recti. In addition, do not use a muscle hook to pull the muscle insertion into the surgical field. Instead, establish exposure of the muscle insertion by use of a limbal traction suture. Finally, do not pull up on the muscle to tent the muscle off the sclera so the muscle can be sutured. Rather, place the Wright grooved hook under the muscle to provide a space for suturing without pulling. One must avoid the temptation of pulling on the muscle, as this is something we were all taught, and routinely do, with standard strabismus surgery.

## Topical Anesthesia Technique for Rectus Muscle Recession

Preoperatively, medicate the patient with a reversible short acting sedative, such as midazolam (Versed). We prefer to have an intravenous line in place and have the patient fully monitored by an anesthesiologist. Topical anesthesia is established by topical tetracaine and lidocaine gel. Topical neosynephirine 2.5% is given to help reduce bleeding. A space is created over the patient's mouth and nose to provide comfortable breathing. Air is circulated via a nasal canula but we try to avoid nasal oxygen to reduce the risk of an oxygen fire. Cautery is also avoided if possible because of the fire risk, and it causes a bad smell for the patient.

Below is a description of topical anesthesia for lateral rectus recession performed on a young man. We have found that the use of midazolam allows us to use topical anesthesia even on that typically difficult and anxious young male!

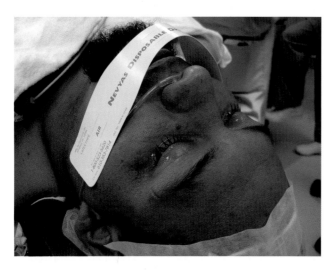

**FIGURE 12.1.** Cardboard arch over the patient's mouth to keep the surgical drapes off the patient and maintain the airway. Nasal canula is in place to supply room air circulation.

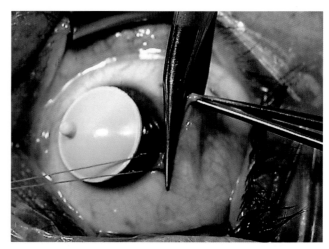

**FIGURE 12.2.** A 6-0 Vicryl traction suture has been placed at the limbus to pull the lateral rectus insertion into the center of the surgical field. A corneal cap covers the pupil so the surgical spotlights do not bother the patient. The limbal incision shown here using the blunt Westcott scissors, along with two radial wing incisions, provides easy access to the muscle without pulling on the muscle.

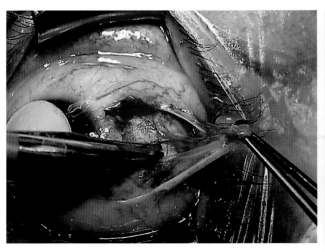
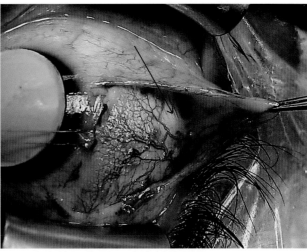

FIGURE 12.3. (A) With the eye held in adduction by the traction suture, mobilize the conjunctiva that overlies the lateral rectus insertion. Free the conjunctiva by blunt and sharp dissection of anterior Tenon's capsule, check ligaments, and intermuscular septum. "Clean" back for only a few millimeters, as extensive dissection does not improve outcomes but increases postoperative scarring. The dissection is performed without a muscle hook pulling on the muscle, as with standard strabismus surgery. (B) The conjunctiva has been mobilized and is being held up off the lateral rectus insertion. The multiple branches of the anterior ciliary artery are seen coming off the lateral rectus. The arrow points to the inferior border of the lateral rectus insertion.

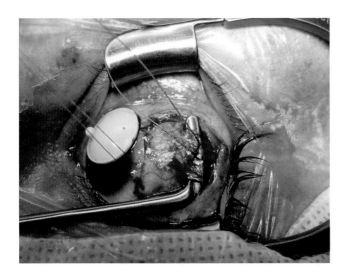
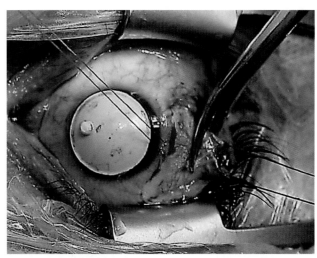

FIGURE 12.4. The Wright grooved hook has been placed behind the lateral rectus muscle to allow suturing of the muscle over the groove in the hook. Do not pull on the hook as this will cause pain. The limbal traction suture holds the eye in position. The grooved hook is only to facilitate suturing the muscle. The photograph shows the central security knot in place. Suture the muscle in the usual manner with a central security knot and locking bites at each edge of the muscle.

FIGURE 12.5. With the hook removed, the muscle sutures are gently pulled up so the tendon can be cut off the sclera with the Westcott scissors. Alternatively, you can leave the muscle hook in place to remove the tendon. This part of the surgery may cause some discomfort as it requires pulling on the muscle. Once the muscle is removed and the muscle tension is relaxed the patient will be comfortable.

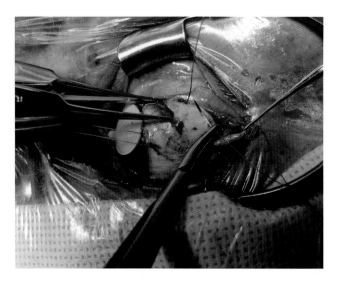

**FIGURE 12.6.** The eye is stabilized with locking forceps and the muscle is secured to sclera with scleral needle passes. Locking forceps are placed on the sclera and scleral needle passes are made without additional topical anesthesia. The sclera is not pain sensitive and these maneuvers do not cause pain.

**Note:** Some surgeons will use a hang-back technique and tie the muscle with a bow tie knot so the muscle can be adjusted. Topical anesthesia does allow for intraoperative adjustment and immediate assessment of alignment. Except for rare exceptionally complex cases, I prefer the fixed suture technique, as in the past I have often adjusted myself out of a good result. Laurie Christensen from Portland, Oregon substantiates my clinical impression and has reported excellent results in complex thyroid related strabismus cases using the fixed suture technique.[1]

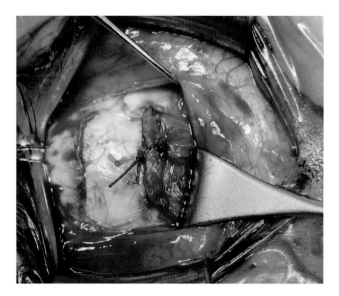

**FIGURE 12.7.** The muscle is in place, recessed posterior to the original scleral insertion.

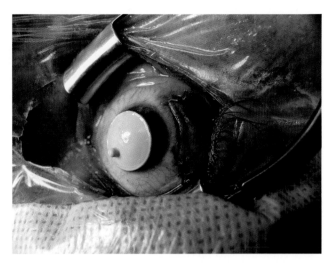

FIGURE 12.8. Suture the conjunctiva back in place as usual. The author prefers a 6-0 plain gut fast absorbing suture. Add an additional dose of topical anesthesia (tetracaine) before suturing the conjunctiva, as the effect of the initial dose may have worn off.

# Reference

1. Gilbert J, Dailey RA, Christensen LE. Characteristics and outcomes of strabismus surgery after orbital decompression for thyroid eye disease. J AAPOS 2005;9:26–30.

# 13  Adjustable Suture Technique

The adjustable suture technique allows for changing the muscle position in the immediate postoperative period while the patient is awake. Therefore, this technique has the theoretical advantage of allowing fine tuning of ocular alignment. Unfortunately, fine tuning must be done within the first 24 to 48 hours of the procedure, when the muscle function has not completely returned and the patient may still have residual effects of anesthesia. Muscle adjustment requires pulling on the muscle and is often uncomfortable for the patient. Another shortcoming of adjustable sutures is the lack of direct scleral fixation and late changes in muscle position. Ludwig and Chow described the association of stretched scar as a cause of late overcorrection after rectus muscle recession.[1] (see Prevention of Late Overcorrection on page 148). Alternatively, large recessions (especially on the lateral rectus) can result in an undercorrection, as the muscle will creep forward. For most "normal" rectus muscles, the maximum you can hang back a muscle on an adjustable suture is 6 mm. A "tight" muscle, however, can retract back for large recessions. Because of these concerns, and the success of the fixed suture technique, this author prefers using a fixed suture with direct scleral fixation. It is important to note that throughout the great career of the late Dr. Marshall Parks, he did not use the adjustable suture technique.

Even though adjustable sutures have a limited role in my practice, there are situations in which they can be helpful. Some of the most important indications for an adjustable suture are complicated strabismus cases, including paralytic strabismus, and large-angle strabismus. In these situations, the standard tables for surgical measurements do not apply, and results with the fixed suture technique may be unpredictable. The adjustable suture, as described below, is used exclusively for rectus muscle recessions.

## Patient Selection

Patient selection is crucial for successful implementation of the adjustable suture technique. The adjustment procedure is somewhat uncomfortable and can evoke substantial anxiety. There is no specific age limit for the use of adjustable sutures, but patients younger than 15 years of age are often anxious about medical procedures and, unless a child is exceptional, the procedure should be limited to cooperative adult patients.

The Q-tip test is a simple and accurate way of identifying patients who will be suitable for the adjustment procedure. This test consists of touching a cotton swab to the medial or lateral aspect of the bulbar conjunctiva. If the patient is able to tolerate manipulation of the bulbar conjunctiva without

136

topical anesthesia, then the patient should do well with the adjustment procedure. It is important to advise patients that the adjustment procedure will be uncomfortable, and avoid patients who are fearful of the procedure or fail the Q-tip test.

## Initial Anesthesia Considerations

The initial surgery and suture placement can be performed under local or general anesthesia. When local anesthesia is used, avoid long-acting agents like bupivicaine (Marcaine) because the akinesia can last for 12 hours or longer, possibly interfering with the adjustment procedure. Local injection of lidocaine with hyaluronidase, and without epinephrine, is preferred, because lidocaine akinesia lasts approximately 2 to 3 hours. Wait for at least 4 to 5 hours after the initial surgery before performing the adjustment to be sure the effects of the lidocaine have completely worn off.

## Surgical Techniques

The operation is performed in two stages. In the first stage, surgery is performed under general or local anesthesia, and the muscle is placed on a suture in such a way that the muscle position can be adjusted later. The second stage, or adjustment stage, is performed when the patient is fully awake or after the local anesthetic has worn off and the muscle's function has returned to normal. During this stage, the muscle is adjusted to properly align the eyes and the suture is permanently tied in place.

### *Limbal versus Fornix Approach*

Limbal surgery provides broad exposure, facilitating suture adjustment. Unless the fornix incision is your procedure of choice, learn the limbal adjustment surgery first. Also, beware of using the fornix technique on patients older than 40 years of age, because older patients have friable conjunctiva that may tear during the stretching maneuvers associated with fornix surgery. Advantages of the fornix approach include a hidden incision underneath the lid, patient comfort, and minimal scarring.

## Limbal Approach: Sliding Noose Technique

### *Left Lateral Rectus Recession (Surgeon's View)*

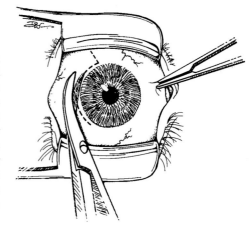

FIGURE 13.1. A limbal incision is made. The muscle is secured and disinserted from sclera in the routine fashion. Make the incision directly in front of the muscle, with either a single or double wing incision. A single wing incision in the inferior temporal quadrant is shown in the drawing. At this point the adjustable suture technique is as follows:

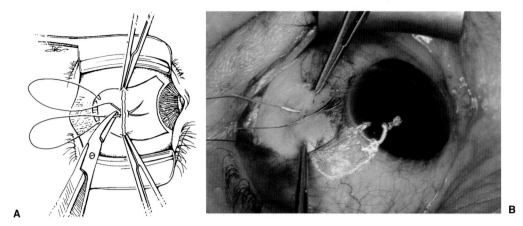

**FIGURE 13.2.** **(A)** The insertion is identified and grasped with two 0.5 Castroviejo locking forceps. Spatula needles from the double-arm sutures are passed perpendicular to the scleral insertion line through half-thickness sclera, securing the muscle to the sclera. The scleral bites are centered on the insertion line. The first needle should be left in place while the second needle is directed with a slight slant toward the first, so they exit the sclera touching (i.e., crossed-swords technique). **(B)** The photograph shows the crossed-swords technique with the needles directed perpendicular to the scleral insertion line. Note: 6-0 Vicryl is preferred for the sliding noose technique as it leaves a smaller knot than 5-0 Vicryl after "tie-off" at the end of the case.

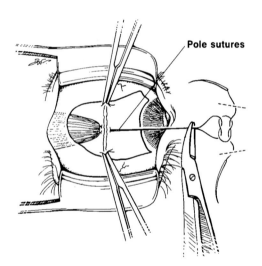

**FIGURE 13.3.** Needles are removed from the sclera, and the sutures are pulled up so the muscle is drawn anteriorly to abut the scleral insertion. A needle holder is clamped across the two sutures approximately 7 mm off the sclera, and the two sutures are tied together in a square knot over the needle holder. This maneuver places the sutures at equal length, and these joined sutures are called the pole sutures. The muscle can be advanced or recessed by pulling or releasing the pole sutures.

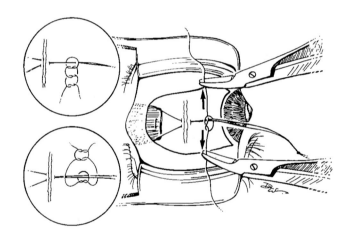

**FIGURE 13.4.** A stop is needed to secure the pole suture to a desired position and to keep the muscle from retracting posteriorly. The stop is created by tying a separate piece of 6-0 coated Vicryl suture (approximately 5 cm long) around the pole sutures with a square knot of three single overhand throws (*upper inset*). This knot forms a noose around the pole sutures and must be extremely tight, because friction from the noose provides the force that holds the muscle in the desired location. Avoid a loose noose by tying an extremely tight single overhand knot as the first throw. A double throw places too much suture around the pole sutures, which prevents adequate tightening of the first knot. A modification that helps to ensure a tight noose is the double-sided square knot (*lower inset*). Each throw is a single overhand knot, but the second and third throw of the knot are on the opposite side of the pole suture from the first throw. The double-sided square knot is the author's preference because it provides a consistently tight noose preventing inadvertent slippage of the noose.

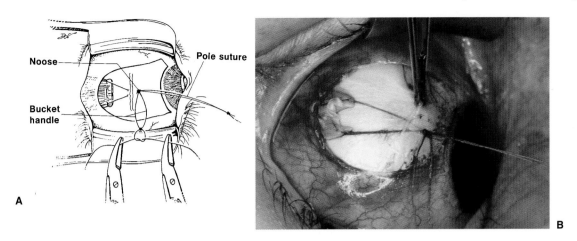

**FIGURE 13.5.** (**A**) The ends of the noose suture are tied together to provide a bucket handle for manipulation of the noose during adjustment. (**B**) The photograph shows a muscle slung back, with the noose acting as a stop against the sclera.

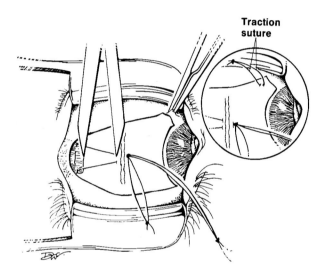

**FIGURE 13.6.** The amount of recession can be measured by releasing the pole sutures and rotating the eye away from the recessed muscle, so that the muscle retracts posteriorly, stopping as the noose contacts the sclera. A single arm 6-0 Vicryl suture (a piece cut from the pole suture) on a S-29 spatula needle can be placed intrascleral near the limbus, to be used as a traction suture during the adjustment procedure (*inset*).

After the surgery is completed, the sutures are folded over the upper lid, stuck down with ophthalmic ointment, and covered with a patch to protect the sutures from inadvertently being pulled. The patch eliminates preadjustment diplopia and has the advantage of covering the sutures so the patient does not inadvertently pull them, mistaking the suture for a hair. An alternative is to place steri-strips over the sutures and tape them to the forehead or cheek. This is useful if bilateral adjustable sutures are employed so both eyes are not patched.

# Adjustment Procedure

*Muscle Advancement*

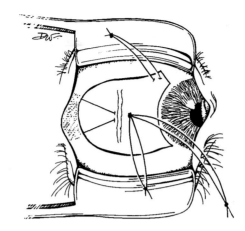

**FIGURE 13.7.** A muscle that has been overre-cessed and needs advancing.

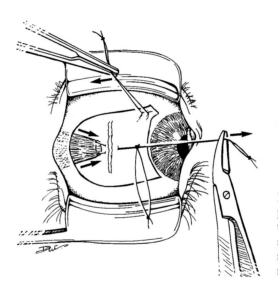

**FIGURE 13.8.** Muscle advancement is accomplished by pulling up on the pole sutures to draw the muscle forward (anteriorly), while the traction suture is pulled to rotate the globe toward the muscle. This maneuver advances the muscle and moves the noose suture up and off the sclera.

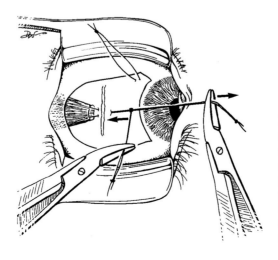

**FIGURE 13.9.** After the muscle is advanced and the noose pulled off the sclera, the pole sutures are stabilized with a needle holder and the noose slid posteriorly to the sclera. This sets the muscle position and prevents posterior slippage of the pole sutures. If the eyes are in proper alignment, the pole sutures are tied together and the excess suture removed (see Tie-Off section later in this chapter).

*Increasing the Recession*

**FIGURE 13.10.** In this situation, the muscle is not recessed enough and needs further recession.

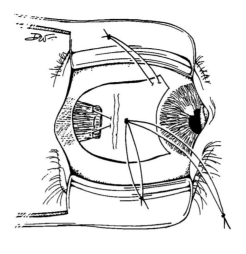

**FIGURE 13.11.** The first maneuver for increasing a recession seems paradoxical, because it consists of advancing the muscle. The pole sutures are pulled forward, and the eye is rotated toward the muscle to lift the noose off the sclera.

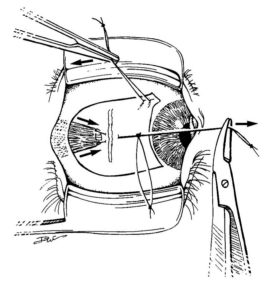

**FIGURE 13.12.** A needle holder is used to grasp and stabilize the exposed pole sutures below the noose. With a second needle holder, the noose is grasped and moved along the pole sutures, away from the muscle, increasing the recession.

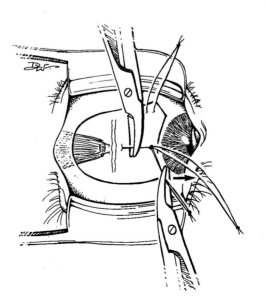

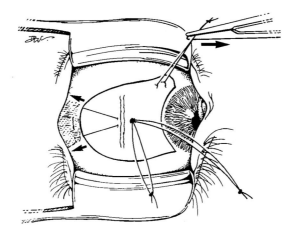

**FIGURE 13.13.** Once the noose is adjusted, the pole sutures are released, and the patient is asked to look toward the recessed muscle. As the muscle contracts, the eye is rotated in the opposite direction, retracting the muscle posteriorly and forcing the noose to firmly against the sclera. It is important that no slack is present after adjustment, because suture slack can lead to late muscle slippage and overcorrection. If the eyes are in proper alignment, the sutures are tied in place (see Tie-Off section below).

*Tie-Off*

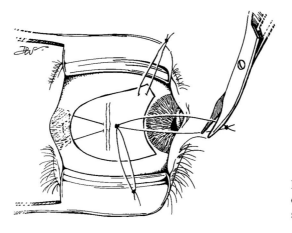

**FIGURE 13.14.** After the muscle is adjusted, one of the pole sutures is cut to separate the pole sutures.

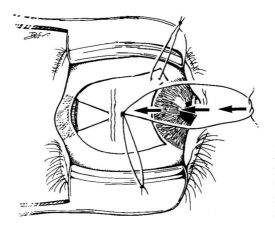

**FIGURE 13.15.** The separated pole sutures are tied firmly together in three overhand knots over the noose to permanently secure the muscle. Do not pull up on the pole sutures during tie-down, as this may change the position of the muscle.

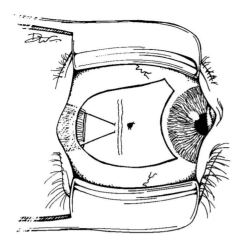

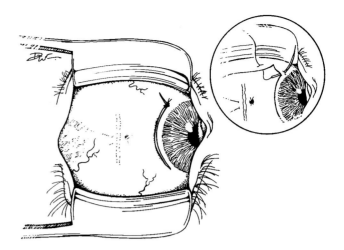

**FIGURE 13.16.** The excess pole sutures and noose bucket handle are removed close to the noose with the Westcott scissors. The knot is shown lying directly on sclera. If a traction suture is present, it can now be removed.

**FIGURE 13.17.** The conjunctival wing incision is closed with a 6-0 plain gut suture (*see inset*). A small conjunctival recession is acceptable, but be sure that the knot is covered. An optional technique is preplacing the conjunctival sutures during the primary surgery and tying them off after the final adjustment.

## Fornix Approach: Sliding Noose Technique

The fornix approach provides an excellent cosmetic result and is very comfortable for the patient. Learning the technique is well worth the effort. To avoid redundancy, details regarding fornix incision and muscle isolation have already been provided in Chapter 11. The adjustable suture apparatus and technique for the fornix approach are essentially the same as the limbal approach using a noose to hold the muscle position. The following technique using a subconjunctival traction suture was developed by the author.[2]

*Left Lateral Rectus Recession*

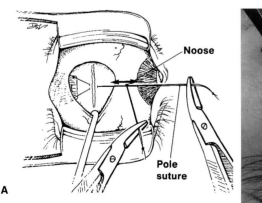

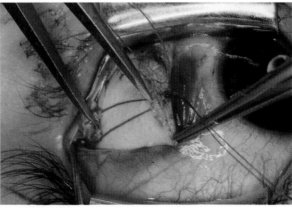

**FIGURE 13.18.** **(A)** Using the fornix incision, the lateral rectus muscle has been sutured to the scleral insertion. The figure shows the noose around the pole sutures. The noose holds the pole sutures in place (see Figure 13.4). Sliding the noose up and down the pole suture adjusts the amount of recession. **(B)** The photograph demonstrates measurement of rectus muscle recession. The muscle is slung back posteriorly with the pole sutures taut, as the eye is rotated away from the muscle. Notice that the noose resting on the sclera prevents the pole sutures from retracting posteriorly. A caliper is used to measure the amount of recession. A locking forceps is left on the superior end of the scleral insertion to hold conjunctiva off the surgical field.

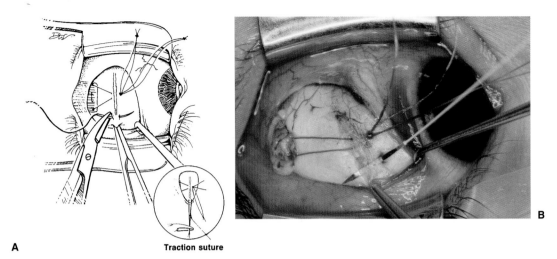

**FIGURE 13.19.** **(A)** The key to the fornix adjustable suture technique is to provide adequate exposure during the adjustment stage. A scleral traction suture that also retracts the conjunctiva accomplishes this goal. A traction suture is placed through half-thickness sclera just superior to the superior end of the insertion line. Pulling up on the traction suture retracts conjunctiva to expose the pole sutures and noose during the adjustment procedure (*see inset*). **(B)** The photograph shows a 5-0 Mersilene single arm suture on a spatula needle being passed at the superior end of the insertion line. Two small Stevens hooks retract the conjunctiva superiorly to provide exposure for the pass.

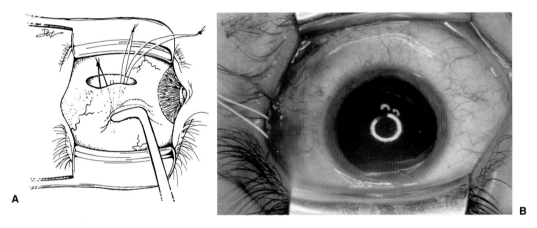

**FIGURE 13.20.** **(A)** The conjunctiva is replaced by pushing the conjunctiva posteriorly toward the fornix with the small Stevens hook. **(B)** The eye at the end of surgery with the sutures exiting the conjunctival incision. After the lid speculum is removed, the sutures are draped over the upper lid and covered with a semipressure patch.

*Adjustment*

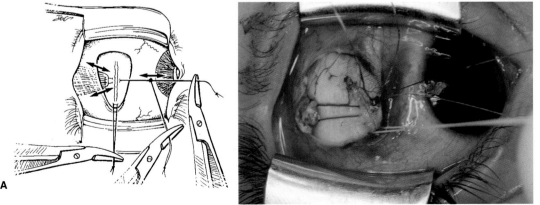

*Tie-Down*

**FIGURE 13.22.** The pole sutures are separated and tied down on top of the noose resting on the sclera. Do not pull up on the pole sutures while tying the pole sutures together, because this can advance the muscle. Three throws are placed over the noose.

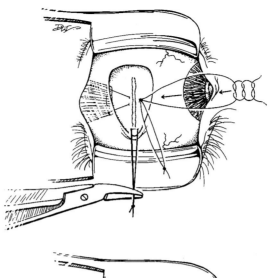

**FIGURE 13.23.** Excess pole sutures and the bucket handle of the noose are removed by cutting the suture close to the knot overlying the noose. Be careful not to cut off the knot or the noose! The traction suture is the last suture to be removed as shown in the drawing.

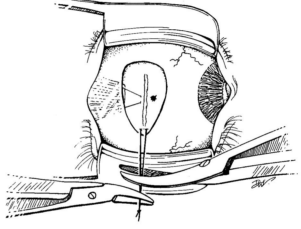

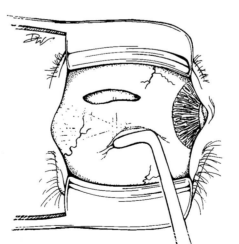

**FIGURE 13.24.** Conjunctiva is pushed over the knot and noose with a small Stevens hook. Surgical closure of conjunctiva is optional.

**FIGURE 13.21. (A)** Pull the conjunctival traction suture superiorly to simultaneously retract the conjunctiva over the noose and stabilize the globe. Once exposed, the noose can be adjusted as described for the limbal approach (see Figures 13.11 to 13.17). **(B)** The traction suture being used to stabilize the globe while retracting the conjunctiva to expose the noose. Notice that the muscle sutures are taut and the noose is firmly against sclera. Make sure there is no slack along the muscle sutures after adjustment. Suture slack can cause changes in the muscle position after adjustment and late postoperative drift.

## Bow-Tie Technique

An alternative to the sliding noose adjustable suture apparatus is the "bow-tie" technique. The rectus muscle is exposed and secured to the sclera in the same manner as previously described for the sliding noose adjustable suture technique, limbal approach. After the pole sutures have been passed through the scleral insertion, they are tied together in a single loop bow-tie.

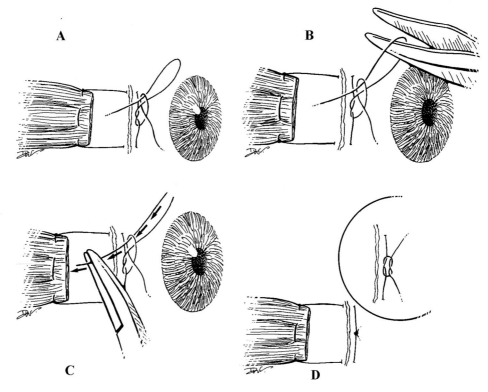

**FIGURE 13.25.** (**A**) Diagram of rectus muscle secured with 6-0 coated Vicryl suture and secured to the scleral insertion by a single loop bow-tie. This knot consists of a single overhand knot followed by a second overhand knot which is left in a single loop. This single loop bow-tie can be untied in order to adjust the position of the muscle. When adjusting the muscle position, make sure that each pole of the muscle is recessed to the same length. (**B**) After the muscle is appropriately adjusted, the bow is tied off by first cutting the loop. (**C**) Then carefully withdraw the cut suture, leaving the knot in place. Do not undo the bow to tie the second throw, as this can lead to muscle slippage. (**D**) The square knot is in place, joining the pole sutures.

## Pearls for Postoperative Adjustment

### Adjustment

The adjustment procedure must be performed within 24 to 48 hours after the initial surgery, while the muscle is freely mobile. Later adjustments are extremely difficult or impossible because the muscle rapidly adheres to the globe. Strong sedatives before adjustment should be avoided because sedation influences eye position. If medication is needed before the adjustment procedure, Tylenol with codeine is preferred. Excellent anesthesia can be obtained by the use of topical tetracaine applied by a moistened cotton swab placed directly over the conjunctiva in the area of the suture. Semi-sterile conditions are sufficient for the adjustment procedure. The patient should wear full optical correction when assessing ocular alignment during the adjustment procedure, to ensure proper image clarity and control of accommodation.

*Anticipating Postoperative Drift*

The goal of the adjustment procedure is not necessarily to place the eyes in an orthotropic position on the first day after surgery, but to obtain alignment that will lead to straight eyes for the long term. The key to successful adjustment is to anticipate postoperative drift. Generally, patients undergoing bilateral recessions show recovery of muscle function, and a good rule of thumb is to adjust these patients to a small overcorrection. This rule holds true for standard recessions, but caution should be observed when performing supermaximal recessions (i.e., >7.5 mm medial rectus and >8.5 mm lateral rectus). In these cases, there is often a permanent weakening effect with a postoperative drift toward overcorrection rather than muscle recovery. Monocular recession-resection procedures, on the other hand, are associated with minimal postoperative drift. When adjusting a patient with sensory esotropia or sensory exotropia, it is important to remember that the adjustment should be based on cosmetic appearance or Krimsky test, rather than on the alternate cover test. Table 13.1 shows recommendations for alignment on the day after surgery for common horizontal strabismus.

TABLE 13.1. Alignment the Day after Surgery

| Diagnosis | Surgery | Adjust to (prism diopters) |
| --- | --- | --- |
| Intermittent exotropia | Recess-resect | ET 4–6 |
| | Bilateral recession | ET 6–8 |
| Sensory exotropia* | Recess-resect | ET 4–6 |
| Adult esotropia | Recess-resect | Ortho |
| | Bimedial recessions | XT 2–4 |
| Accommodative esotropia (fusional potential) | Bimedial recessions | XT 4–6 |
| Sensory esotropia* | Recess-resect | Ortho |

*Always perform monocular surgery on the amblyopic eye.*

## Complications

Fortunately, complications following the adjustable suture technique are rare. One might expect a high incidence of postoperative infection or cellulitis because the adjustment procedure is performed in the office under semisterile conditions. Postoperative infections, however, are no more frequent than with standard fixed suture techniques. A minor complication of practical importance is the persistence and irritation of a suture knot after adjustment and tie down. If an irritating knot persists, it can be safely removed as soon as 3 weeks after surgery without subsequent muscle slippage. Other concerns are the oculocardiac reflex and possible brady-cardia associated with muscle manipulations. Overall, the adjustable suture technique is a safe procedure for treatment of complicated strabismus.

## Preventing Late Overcorrection

Late overcorrection after adjustable suture surgery is most likely due to suture dissolution before the muscle tendon fully adheres to sclera! This complication of late overcorrection is most frequently seen after surgery on a tight rectus muscle such as medial rectus and inferior rectus in thyroid related strabismus. The technique to avoid late overcorrection is to secure the muscle with a nonabsorbable suture after adjustment and tie-off. A 5-0 Mersilene suture is used to secure the muscle edge to the sclera posterior to the Vicryl suture.

## References

1. Ludwig I, Chow A. Scar remodeling after strabismus surgery. J AAPOS 2000;4:326–333.
2. Wright KW, McVey JH. Conjunctival retraction suture for fornix adjustable strabismus surgery. Arch Ophthalmol 1991;109:138–141.

# 14  Rectus Muscle Tightening Procedures

## Rectus Muscle Resection

The two most useful rectus muscle tightening procedures are the rectus muscle resection and the rectus muscle plication. Rectus muscle tucking has not proven reliable, as it tends to loosen over time. A tuck is a muscle-to-muscle union. Because the muscle fibers are longitudinal and the transverse fibers are weak, the sutures tend to pull out and slip. The rectus muscle plication, however, involves securing posterior muscle to sclera, and this procedure is as stable as a resection.

Muscle resections can be done as a single or double-suture procedure. The single-suture technique is preferred by the author because it is simple, fast, and accomplishes the same anatomic goals as the double suture technique. One key to the single-suture technique is to place a security knot in the center of the muscle to prevent unraveling of the suture if one of the sutures is inadvertently cut or broken. Proponents of the double-suture technique prefer two sutures for greater security against a lost muscle and for better support of the middle of the muscle. Plications and resections can be performed through either a fornix or limbal incision.

## Single Suture Resection: Fornix Approach

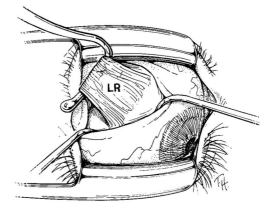

FIGURE 14.1.  (Surgeon's view) The left lateral rectus muscle is isolated in the standard manner through a fornix incision. A posterior dissection, including the intermuscular septum and check ligaments, is performed to approximately 3 mm posterior to the planned muscle resection (see Figures 10.9 and 10.10 for posterior dissection technique). The anterior Tenon's capsule is removed in front of the muscle to expose bare sclera.

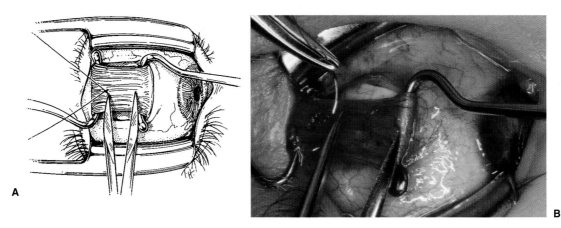

**FIGURE 14.2.** **(A)** Two large Jameson hooks are inserted under the muscle belly. One hook is placed at the insertion (handle directed nasally), and the other is placed posteriorly deep in the fornix (handle directed temporally). Keep the posterior hook against sclera and avoid the temptation to pull the hook up to obtain more muscle. Pulling the hook off sclera does not gain access to posterior muscle; this only stretches the anterior muscle, which is already exposed. A security knot is placed through the center of the muscle belly. **(B)** The photograph shows that the calipers are placed at the center of the Jameson hook and posteriorly, to mark the location of the security knot. A 5-0 Vicryl double arm suture is used to secure a central 2 mm area of muscle (full-muscle thickness). Notice that the needle is placed approximately 0.5 mm to 1 mm posterior to the desired resection point. This places the security knot behind the resection point, which helps protect the knot. The sutures are tied together in a tight square knot. If one of the sutures inadvertently breaks, this knot will secure the muscle and prevent the suture from completely unraveling.

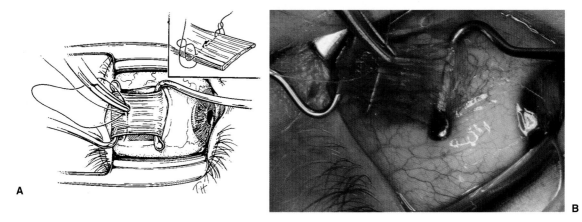

**FIGURE 14.3.** **(A)** One of the needles connected to the security knot is passed at half-muscle thickness, entering just anterior to the knot. This pass extends half thickness until it exits at the muscle edge. A full-thickness locking bite is then placed through 2 mm of the muscle edge, directly behind the half-thickness suture. Using the other end of the suture, the same suture pass is performed on the other half of the muscle to secure both sides of the muscle. The *inset* shows the suture path with locking bites at each edge of the muscle, and a security knot in the center of the muscle. **(B)** The companion photograph shows the needle being passed at half-thickness through the superior aspect of the lateral rectus muscle, just anterior to the security knot. Keep the needle pass parallel to the hooks, because the tendency is to slant the pass anteriorly, reducing the resection.

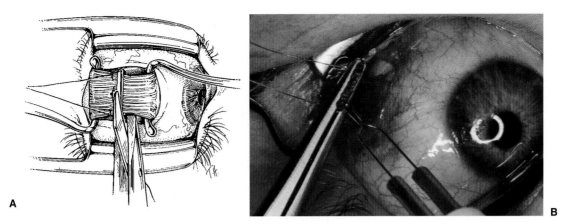

**FIGURE 14.4.** **(A)** The muscle has been secured with 5-0 Vicryl suture, by placing locking bites at each edge of the muscle, as well as a central security knot. The muscle is then cross-clamped with a Hartman clamp, anterior to the sutures. Next the muscle is excised anterior to the Hartman clamp, flush to the surface of the clamp. **(B)** The photograph shows cautery being applied to the muscle stump. Note the sutures being pulled posteriorly in order to avoid cautery. Be careful, because the sutures will melt and weaken if they get close to the cautery. After cautery, the muscle is released from the Hartman clamp. **Note:** The author does not routinely clamp and cauterize the lateral rectus muscle, as it does not hemorrhage significantly after being resected.

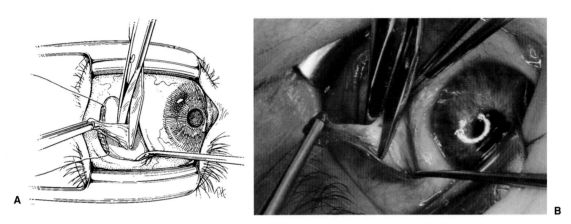

**FIGURE 14.5.** **(A)** Remove the muscle stump close to sclera so that the scleral insertion can be directly visualized. A residual muscle stump gives false security because sutures can easily loosen if passed through residual tendon fibers rather than sclera. **(B)** The muscle stump being removed from its scleral insertion.

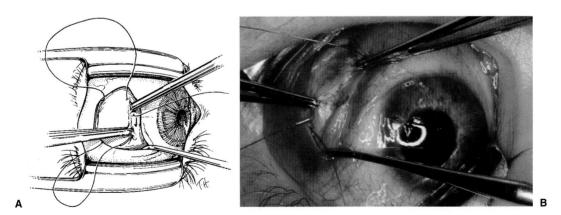

**FIGURE 14.6.** **(A)** The scleral insertion is secured with two 0.5 Castroviejo locking forceps. Forceps are placed 1 mm inside the ends of the scleral insertion line. This provides space at the end of the scleral insertion for needle placement. The muscle is secured to the original insertion with deep scleral bites at the insertion line. The scleral thickness in front of the muscle insertion is at least twice as thick as the sclera behind the insertion line. It is important to make deep scleral passes so that the suture does not cut through the sclera while pulling the muscle up into position. A needle is shown being passed superior to a locking forceps. **(B)** The companion photograph shows the needle passing through the superior pole of anterior sclera. Notice the deep pass, which is necessary to secure the resected muscle. The locking forceps are "doing the splits," with the lower locking forceps reflected nasally and the superior forceps temporally, allowing clear visualization of the scleral pass. A similar scleral pass is made inferiorly.

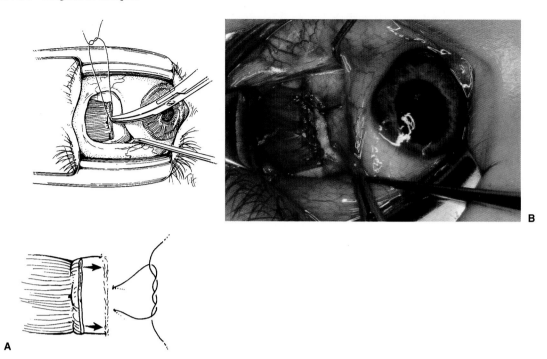

**FIGURE 14.7.** **(A)** The muscle is advanced to the scleral insertion by gently, but firmly, pulling on the sutures. Do not pull up on the sutures; pull parallel to the scleral tunnel to avoid tearing sclera and pulling the suture out of the sclera (similar to a cheese-wire cutting cheese). Tie the sutures together with a double-throw overhand knot, and advance the muscle so both poles are firmly against sclera (shown in close-up drawing of sutures on the facing page). Tighten the knot, and clamp the knot with a needle holder to keep the knot from slipping. Tie the next overhand knot directly over the needle holder. Do not remove the needle holder until the second knot is tightly in place. This technique is analogous to putting your finger on the knot when tying a bow on a package. Three overhand knots should be placed for security. **(B)** The photograph shows the end result, with the muscle against the scleral insertion line. Notice no central sag, even though surgery was done with a single suture technique. The key is to splay out the muscle widely, providing a taut anterior muscle line.

## Double-Suture Resection

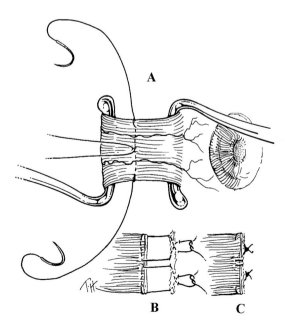

**FIGURE 14.8.** **(A)** In the diagram of the double-suture resection technique, two Jameson hooks are used to place the muscle on stretch, and to access the posterior muscle. Two 5-0 coated Vicryl double arm sutures with spatula needles are used to secure the muscle. The first suture is passed from the center of the muscle toward the edge of the muscle at half thickness. A 2 mm full thickness locking bite is used to secure the edge of the muscle. The second double arm suture is passed in an identical manner in the opposite direction. Once the muscle is secured, the anterior muscle is resected in the standard fashion (see previous section on Rectus Muscle Recession). **(B)** The resected muscle is secured to the scleral insertion by four scleral passes. The two central passes should be performed close together with approximately 1 mm to 2 mm of separation. Double armed sutures are tied together with three overhand knots. **(C)** Final result of the double-suture technique with two double arm sutures tied anterior to the scleral insertion. Note that the center of the muscle is supported by two scleral passes.

## Wright Plication: Rectus Muscle–Scleral Plication (Vessel Sparing)

Another procedure for tightening the rectus muscle is the rectus muscle–scleral plication. A muscle-to-sclera plication was developed by the author. It consists of securing posterior muscle, like in a single suture resection. Instead of resecting the anterior muscle, the sutures are passed through the sclera at the insertion, thereby folding the muscle. Plications have some distinct advantages, including preservation of anterior ciliary vessels, safety, as there is virtually no chance of a lost muscle, and reversibility, by cutting the suture. The author has studied anterior segment blood flow after the plication procedure and found it to reliably preserve anterior ciliary circulation.[1,2] The plication should be strongly considered if multiple rectus muscles are being operated on in the same eye and anterior segment ischemia is a concern.

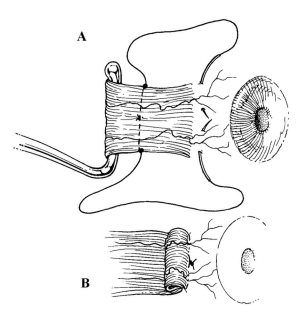

FIGURE 14.9. (A) The muscle is secured with a 5-0 Vicryl double-arm suture with spatula needles. Place the sutures through posterior muscle at the same location as you would for a rectus muscle resection based on the standard charts. The needles are passed through half thickness muscle, starting in the center of the muscle, aiming perpendicular to the muscle fibers, toward the edge of the muscle. A central security knot is optional because the muscle is not being transected. A 2 mm locking bite is then placed at the edge of the muscle. An identical pass is performed on both sides of the muscle. Avoid anterior ciliary arteries; anterior ciliary arteries lie superficial to the muscle in this area and can be avoided by passing the suture deep to the vessels. If a vessel is in the way of a locking bite, it can be gently moved aside with a smooth instrument, such as a small Stevens hook. The needles are passed through the sclera just anterior to the muscle insertion. Again, avoid impaling anterior ciliary vessels. Anterior to the muscle, there are multiple branches of the anterior ciliary vessels, and it is almost impossible to miss them all. The idea is to leave as many of the arterial branches intact as possible. (B) Posterior muscle is advanced by pulling on the double arm sutures. A double throw overhand knot is secured, and the needle holder pinches the knot so it does not loosen when the second overhand throw is placed. The plication causes a small bulge of tissue that will flatten over 6 weeks and does not present a significant cosmetic problem. **Note:** The plication can be reversed by cutting the suture, but it must be done within 3 days of the surgery or the muscle will have already healed to sclera.

# Left Medial Rectus Plication: Fornix Incision

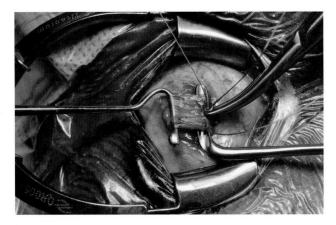

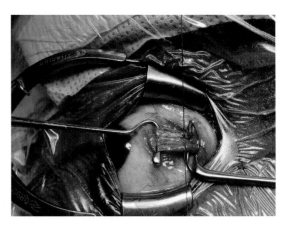

**FIGURE 14.10.** The left medial rectus muscle has been hooked and dissected clear of check ligaments and intermuscular septum through a fornix incision. The Wright grooved hook is placed at the plication site posterior to the insertion. The muscle is secured with a double arm 5-0 Vicryl suture in the standard manner with locking bites at each edge of the muscle. Drawing shows the needle being passed from the center to exit at the edge of the medial rectus muscle.

**FIGURE 14.11.** Two-point fixation with locking bites at each edge of the muscle. To preserve anterior ciliary circulation, a central security knot was not placed.

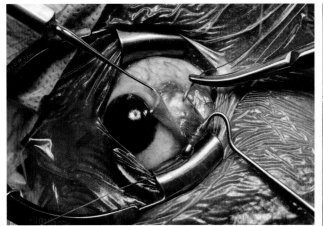

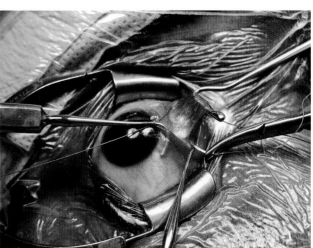

A

B

**FIGURE 14.12. (A)** The needle attached to the muscle is passed 1 mm anterior to the inferior pole of the medial rectus muscle. Make a secure pass, as the muscle will be under tension during the plication. A small Stevens hook is retracting the conjunctiva for exposure of the sclera anterior to the muscle insertion. **(B)** The superior pole needle pass through sclera 1 mm to 2 mm anterior to the medial rectus insertion. Two small Stevens hooks retract the conjunctiva for scleral exposure.

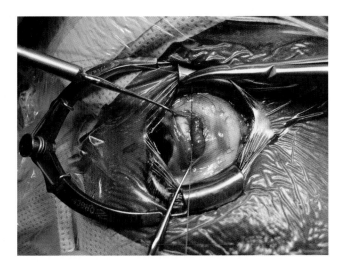

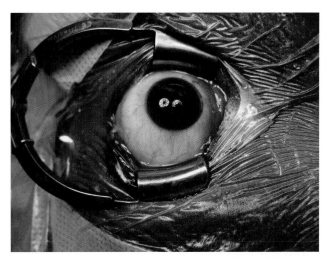

**FIGURE 14.13.** The muscle has been plicated by pulling on the sutures. The technique is to first pull both sutures up to the ceiling then, keeping the sutures tight, secondarily pull down to seat the knot onto sclera. Pull several times until the plication is fully advanced. Once the suture is tight and the muscle plicated, grasp the knot with a needle holder so it will not slip loose during the tying of the knot.

**FIGURE 14.14.** The conjunctiva has been replaced and sutured. Note there is no significant conjunctival lump from the plication.

# References

1. Wright KW, Lanier AB. Effect of a modified rectus tuck on anterior segment circulation in monkeys. J Pediatr Ophthalmol Strab 1991;28:77–81.
2. Park C, Min B, Wright KW. Effect of a modified rectus tuck on anterior ciliary artery perfusion. Korean J Ophthalmol 1991;5:15–25.

# 15 Horizontal Rectus Muscle Offsets and the Y-Splitting Procedure

## Horizontal Rectus Muscle Transpositions for A and V Patterns

Vertical transposition of horizontal muscle insertions is an effective means of collapsing an A or V pattern. This is true only if there is no significant oblique overaction. If oblique overaction is present, appropriate oblique muscle surgery should be performed.

The rationale for vertical transposition is based on the observation that the strength of a horizontal rectus muscle is increased when the eye is vertically rotated in the direction opposite to the direction of its transposed insertion. For example, lowering the insertion of a horizontal rectus muscle improves the effect of this muscle when the eye is in elevation. Conversely, an elevated horizontal rectus muscle insertion produces more effect in depression. Therefore, an esotropic V pattern would best be improved by moving a recessed medial rectus muscle inferiorly, which produces more adduction in up gaze and less in down gaze. Similarly, displacing a resected lateral rectus muscle insertion superiorly decreases its abducting effect in up gaze while increasing the effect in down gaze. The result is a reduction in the size of the pattern deviation. Vertical transpositions of horizontal muscles do not appreciably alter the horizontal alignment in primary position.

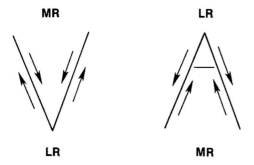

**FIGURE 15.1.** A medial rectus muscle, whether resected, recessed, or simply transposed, is always moved toward the apex of the pattern. Thus, the medial rectus muscle is displaced inferiorly in V patterns and superiorly in A patterns. Conversely, a lateral rectus muscle is moved away from the apex, superiorly for V patterns and inferiorly for A patterns. The magnitude of the transposition usually performed is either half of a tendon width or a full tendon width. The former amount corrects patterns of 10 PD to 25 PD; the latter is used for patterns exceeding 25 PD.

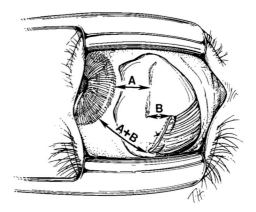

FIGURE 15.2. Full tendon inferior transposition with recession. The most crucial part of the procedure is determining the site for scleral reattachment of the muscle, as it is important not to advance or recess the muscle inappropriately. This is done by measuring the distance to the muscle's new insertion radially from the limbus. For a recession, the planned amount of recession (B) is added to the distance from limbus to the original insertion (A). The surgeon first measures the amount of recession (A + B) from the limbus to the pole of the muscle closest to the original insertion. The suture is passed through the sclera in the standard fashion. The second pole of the muscle is then reattached at the same distance from the limbus (A + B), spreading the muscle poles approximately 8mm apart. The two arms of the suture are then tied together. The reattached muscle's leading edge parallels the curving limbus.

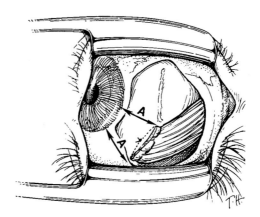

FIGURE 15.3. Full tendon inferior transposition of a resected muscle. The distance to each of the muscle poles from the limbus is the distance from the limbus to the midpoint of the original insertion. The muscle is transposed inferiorly by one tendon width. The muscle poles are spread apart by approximately 8mm.

## Horizontal Rectus Muscle Transpositions for Vertical Strabismus

Moving the medial and lateral rectus muscles up or down is useful for correcting small, comitant vertical deviations that occur in association with horizontal strabismus. In this procedure, the horizontal muscle

insertions of a hypertropic eye are lowered or the horizontal muscle insertions of a hypotropic eye are elevated. Each horizontal muscle is resected
or recessed, as specified by the magnitude of the horizontal deviation.

There is approximately 1 PD of improvement in the vertical deviation
per 1 mm of displacement. This is true when two muscles in the same eye
are transposed in the same direction. Vertical muscle displacements of up
to 8 mm may be readily performed with this technique. It is most useful
when the surgeon is performing monocular recess-resect surgery, in which
both muscles are moved in the same direction (Figure 15.4). It has also
been successfully used for bilateral surgery, in which muscles are moved
in opposite directions. This surgery, however, is not effective if vertical
restrictions (e.g., thyroid orbitopathy) are present.

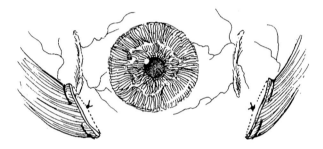

FIGURE 15.4. A one-half tendon width inferior transposition of both horizontal rectus
muscles and recession-resection for correcting horizontal deviation and hypertropia
is shown. The muscle on the left has been resected and infraplaced; the muscle on the
right has been recessed and infraplaced.

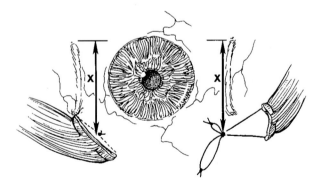

FIGURE 15.5. The diagram shows full tendon width inferior transposition of both
horizontal muscles with an adjustable recession. The method is the same as for the
correction of A and V patterns. The muscles are transposed by the planned number
of millimeters and reattached to the globe, taking all measurements radially from the
limbus to ensure that there is no anterior or posterior placement. This technique may
be performed in conjunction with adjustable suture techniques.

## Rectus Muscle Transpositions for Torsion

Torsional strabismus can be improved by moving vertical rectus muscles nasally or temporally. Nasal placement of the superior rectus causes extorsion (corrects intorsion) while temporal placement causes intorsion (corrects extorsion). The opposite is true for the inferior rectus muscle, with nasal transposition producing intorsion (correcting extorsion) and temporal transposition producing extorsion (correcting intorsion). A transposition of one tendon width (approximately 8 mm) will induce about 4° to 5° of torsion. Most of the torsion effect is seen in the field of action of the transposed muscle. If the superior rectus muscle is transposed nasally 8 mm and the inferior rectus muscle transposed temporally 8 mm, a total of 8° to 10° of extorsion would be induced, thus correcting 10° of intorsion. Horizontal rectus muscle transposition will also produce some torsional changes but less than vertical rectus muscle transpositions. Supraplacement of the medial rectus muscle induces intorsion; infraplacement induces extorsion. The opposite is true for the lateral rectus muscle. Note that it is unusual for a vertical transposition of a horizontal muscle to induce significant torsion.

Most cases of torsional strabismus are caused by oblique dysfunction and, if oblique dysfunction is present, operate on the oblique muscles to correct the torsion. For example, extorsion associated with bilateral superior oblique paresis is usually best handled by bilateral Harada-Ito procedures, not a rectus muscle transposition.

## Y-Splitting of the Lateral Rectus Muscle for Duane's Retraction Syndrome

Y-split of the lateral rectus muscle is employed for patients with Duane's retraction syndrome, who have significant upshoot and downshoot of the eye as it is rotated into adduction (see Chapter 7). If an esotropia is present

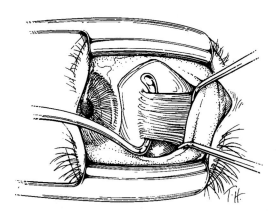

FIGURE 15.6. The lateral rectus muscle is isolated and exposed by removing check ligaments.

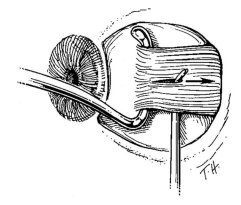

FIGURE 15.7. The muscle is split into two halves for a distance of 14 mm posteriorly from the insertion using a Stevens hook.

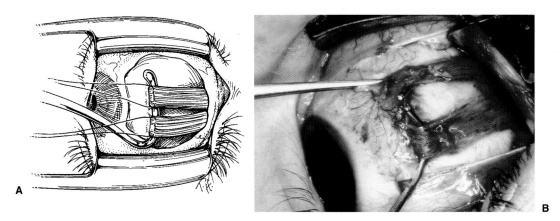

**FIGURE 15.8. (A)** Absorbable sutures are placed through both the upper and lower halves of the insertion, just as in standard strabismus surgery. **(B)** The lateral rectus muscle is split with two Stevens hooks.

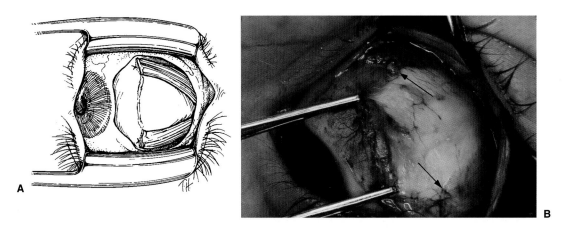

**FIGURE 15.9. (A)** The drawing shows a Y-split of the lateral rectus muscle without recession. The halves of the lateral rectus muscle are reattached to sclera above and below the lateral rectus insertion. The upper portion of the muscle is reattached with its inferior edge adjacent to the superior end of the insertion. The superior border of the upper portion is attached to the sclera, maintaining the same distance from the limbus to the muscle. The inferior half is reattached with its superior border adjacent to the inferior border of the insertion. The inferior edge is then reattached further inferiorly, at the same distance from the limbus as its superior edge. The reattached muscle thus forms a "Y." **(B)** The Y-split lateral rectus muscle with a 4mm recession for an XT Duane's retraction syndrome. The muscle halves can barely be identified above and below white sclera *(arrows)*. The picture emphasizes the breadth of splitting necessary for correcting the upshoot and downshoot associated with Duane's retraction syndrome.

in primary position causing a face turn, then a medial rectus recession is performed with the Y-split of the lateral rectus muscle. For patients with an "XT" Duane's retraction syndrome, the ipsilateral lateral rectus undergoing the Y-splitting should be recessed.

# 16 Transposition Surgery for Rectus Muscle Palsy

Transposition surgery is based on changing the location of the muscle insertion so the muscle pulls the eye in a different direction (i.e., changes the vector of forces). Transposition surgeries can be used to treat a rectus muscle paresis, a lost muscle, A and V patterns (Chapter 15), small vertical tropias (Chapter 15), and torsion (Chapter 15). Three transposition procedures will be described in this chapter: Knapp, Jensen, and Hummelsheim.

## Knapp Procedure

A full-tendon transfer was originally described for the management of double elevator palsy. This procedure, however, can also be used for sixth nerve palsy. The key for successful surgery is symmetrical transposition to avoid induced vertical or horizontal deviations. Extensive posterior dissection to free the muscle of the intermuscular septum and check ligaments is necessary to mobilize the muscle for the tendon transfer. A possible complication of the full-tendon transfer is anterior segment ischemia. The author prefers the Hummelsheim partial-tendon transfer for the treatment of rectus muscle paralysis. (See Chapter 8 for strategies regarding the treatment of paralytic strabismus.)

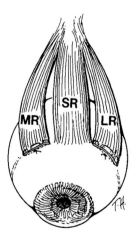

FIGURE 16.1. This diagram shows the Knapp procedure with the medial rectus and lateral rectus muscles transposed superiorly to the insertion of the superior rectus muscle. This procedure has been described for the treatment of double elevator palsy with poor superior rectus muscle function. Two fornix incisions in the superior temporal and superior nasal quadrants provide the best exposure for this procedure.

## Jensen Procedure

The Jensen procedure is a split-tendon transfer with the adjacent muscles tied together, but not disinserted. This procedure has the advantage of preserving the anterior ciliary arteries and diminishing the risk of anterior segment ischemia. Even with the Jensen procedure, however, some vascular compromise occurs, and anterior segment ischemia has been associated with this procedure. Good exposure can be obtained by placing two separate fornix incisions on either side of the paretic muscle.

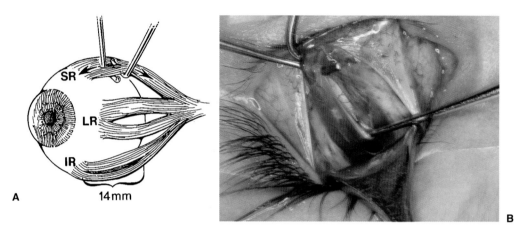

**FIGURE 16.2. (A)** The Jensen procedure used for a left sixth nerve palsy. The superior, inferior and lateral rectus muscles are isolated and cleared of surrounding check ligaments and intermuscular septum. Each of the muscles is split exactly one-half tendon width, with two small Stevens hooks. When splitting the superior and inferior rectus muscles, avoid the anterior ciliary arteries. The muscles should be split at least 12 mm to 14 mm posterior to the insertion. **(B)** The left superior rectus muscle is being split with two small Stevens hooks (surgeon's view). Notice that posterior exposure can be enhanced by removing the lid speculum and inserting a Desmarres retractor under the upper lid.

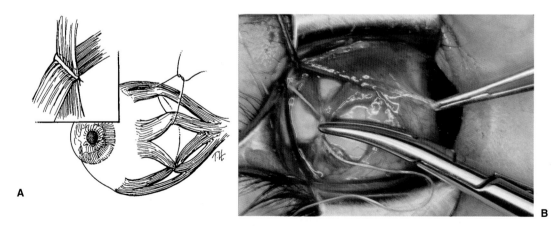

**FIGURE 16.3. (A)** A 5-0 Mersilene suture is laced between adjacent muscle halves (i.e., superior rectus/lateral rectus and inferior rectus/ lateral rectus). These union sutures should be placed at the equator, approximately 12 mm posterior to the limbus. The inset shows the proper muscle union, with a small space between adjoining muscles. The muscles should be tied together in a relatively loose loop to avoid anterior ciliary artery strangulation. The Mersilene suture can be passed through sclera, 12 mm posterior to the limbus, to keep the union posterior. **(B)** The union of superior and lateral rectus muscles with 5-0 Mersilene suture in place. The suture should be tied loosely so that the muscles come together and barely touch. A needle holder is used to hold the first overhand throw of the knot.

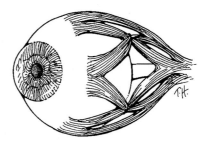

FIGURE 16.4. The final result shows the tendon unions of superior rectus to lateral rectus and inferior rectus to lateral rectus. The posterior location of the union is important. The sutures should be at least 12 mm posterior to the insertions. Anterior union sutures will reduce the effect of the transposition.

## Hummelsheim Procedure

This is a split-tendon transposition designed to preserve anterior ciliary artery perfusion. In contrast to the Jensen procedure, the Hummelsheim procedure can be used for a lost muscle. The Hummelsheim procedure is the author's procedure of choice for a muscle palsy.

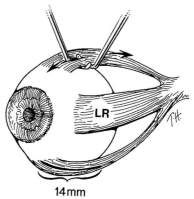

14 mm

FIGURE 16.5. In the Hummelsheim procedure, muscles are isolated, and the check ligaments and intermuscular septum are separated from the muscle in the standard fashion. The muscle is divided exactly in half, and split by blunt dissection with two small Stevens hooks. The splitting of the muscles should extend to approximately 14 mm posterior to the muscle insertion as in the Jensen procedure (Figure 16.2).

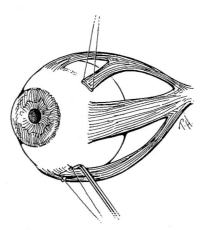

FIGURE 16.6. A 5-0 coated Vicryl double-arm suture is passed through the temporal half of each vertical rectus muscle tendon in the standard fashion, with locking bites on each edge of the muscle. The sutured muscles are disinserted with Westcott scissors.

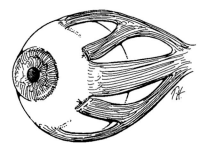

**FIGURE 16.7.** Muscle halves from the superior and inferior recti are transposed and sutured to sclera adjacent to the lateral rectus muscle insertion. Note that the transposed muscle halves insert in line with the lateral rectus insertion.

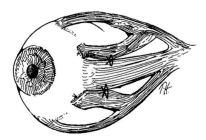

**FIGURE 16.8.** This drawing shows the muscle union Wright modification of the Hummelsheim procedure (see modifications below). With this modification the transposed vertical rectus muscle halves are sutured to the lateral rectus muscle approximately 5mm to 6mm posterior to the lateral rectus insertion, increasing the effect of the transposition.

### Modifications of Transpositions

Three modifications of the Hummelsheim procedure, which increase the effect of the transposition, are listed below. The author prefers the muscle union.

### Brooks Resection Modification (Augmented Hummelsheim)

This procedure consists of resecting 4mm to 6mm of the transposed rectus muscle halves. Resecting some of the transposed muscle halves enhances the transposition by increasing the leash effect.[1]

### Foster Modification (Lateral Scleral Fixation)

A lateral fixation suture of 5-0 Dacron polyester filament was placed in the sclera 16mm posterior to the limbus and adjacent to the lateral rectus muscle,[2] incorporating one fourth of the transposed vertical rectus muscle.

### Wright Modification (Muscle Union)

The muscle union modification consists of suturing the transposed muscle halves to the paretic muscle (Figure 16.8). This directly increases paretic muscle tension and keeps the posterior part of the transposed muscle lateral, thus lateralizing the force vector. This modification is very effective in increasing lateral forces. The author prefers using the Hummelsheim with the muscle union modification over the full tendon transposition (Knapp procedure) because the modified Hummelsheim procedure spares anterior ciliary vessels, thus reducing the risk of anterior segment ischemia. The muscle union modification was described by this author in the second edition of this book.

## Complications

Anterior segment ischemia is always a possibility in transposition surgery. Split-tendon procedures such as the Jensen and Hummelsheim lessen the risks, but even these procedures have been associated with anterior segment ischemia. The best strategy is to preserve as many anterior ciliary arteries as possible. A limbal conjunctival incision disrupts local vessels and may increase the risk of anterior segment ischemia, suggesting that the fornix incision may be preferable.

Transposition procedures can induce unwanted deviations if there is asymmetric muscle placement. In split-tendon procedures, it is important to split and transpose the muscle equally to prevent inadvertent deviations.

## References

1. Brooks SE, Olitsky SE, deB Ribeiro G. Augmented Hummelsheim procedure for paralytic strabismus. J Pediatr Ophthalmol Strabismus 2000;37:189–195.
2. Foster RS, Vertical muscle transposition augmented with lateral fixation. J AAPOS 1997;1:20–30.

# 17  Inferior Oblique Muscle Weakening Procedures

Over the past years, the management of inferior oblique overaction has improved substantially. Historically, inferior oblique surgery was considered extremely difficult and fraught with complications, such as fat adherence, ciliary nerve damage with pupillary dilatation, and intraoperative hemorrhage. The late Dr. Marshall Parks pioneered meticulous techniques that all but eliminated these complications. Another important advance has been the anteriorization procedure.

## Quantification of Inferior Oblique Overaction

Selection of the appropriate surgical procedure is based on the amount of inferior oblique dysfunction. Inferior oblique overaction is clinically estimated on a scale of +1 through +4. When performing versions to test for inferior oblique overaction, make sure the abducting eye is fixing, so the adducting fellow eye is free to manifest an "upshoot." Quantify the upshoot by bringing the fixing eye straight across to the lateral canthus, and observe the adducting eye for upshoot (Figure 17.1).

Inferior oblique overaction causes a V pattern–Y subtype with most of the divergence occurring from primary position to up gaze. The final quantification of inferior oblique overaction should be based on the combined characteristics of the degree of upshoot and amount of V pattern.

## Indications for Surgery

The basic rule of thumb is that patients with +2 or more inferior oblique overaction are candidates for an inferior oblique surgery, and those with +1 or less can usually be followed. Patients with minimal inferior oblique overaction, but a significant V pattern (>15 PD), are exceptions to this rule. These patients should be considered for inferior oblique weakening even though versions show minimal inferior oblique overaction.

Primary inferior oblique overaction is usually bilateral and almost always requires bilateral surgery. In cases of asymmetric overaction, bilateral surgery should be performed, even when one eye displays only +1 overaction, to avoid unmasking the minimal overaction. If amblyopia is present (greater than 2 Snellen lines difference), it is safer to restrict surgery to the amblyopic eye. In these cases, monocular surgery is sufficient because the sound eye is always fixing and will not manifest an upshoot.

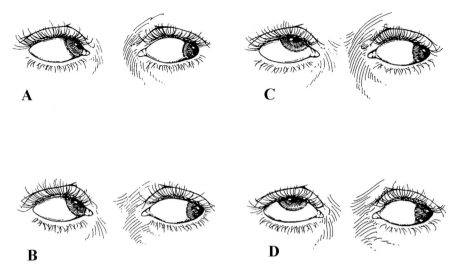

**FIGURE 17.1.** Quantification of upshoot in inferior oblique overaction. Note that the abducting eye (left eye) is the fixing eye and is kept in straight abduction. The adducting eye (right eye) is free to manifest the overaction. One can ensure the abducting eye is fixing by covering the adducting eye with an occluder or your thumb. Look behind the occluder to see the overaction. **(A)** Minimal upshoot (+1) of adducting eye when taken straight across. Upshoot is better seen when the abducting eye is moved up and out. **(B)** Upshoot (+2) of adducting eye is obvious when the abducting eye looks straight across at the lateral canthus. **(C)** Severe upshoot (+3) of adducting eye is seen even with abducting eye in straight abduction. **(D)** Very severe upshoot (+4) of adducting eye is seen as the fixing eye moves straight across into abduction. In addition to a severe upshoot, there will be an abduction movement as the adducting eye is elevated into the field of action of the inferior oblique.

## Making Procedural Choices

Surgical management of inferior oblique muscle overaction is based on weakening or changing the function of the inferior oblique muscle. The most commonly used techniques include myectomy, recession, and anteriorization. Inferior oblique myotomy is not effective, because the cut ends of the muscle inevitably reunite or scar to sclera, causing residual inferior oblique overaction. Myectomy weakens the inferior oblique, as removing a portion of muscle reduces the chance of local reattachment (Figure 17.2A).

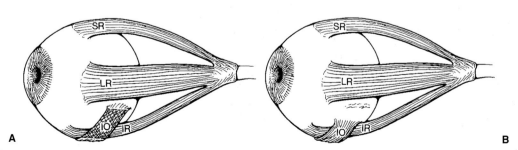

**FIGURE 17.2.** **(A)** Myectomy. Hatch marks represent the portion of the temporal muscle removed in the myectomy procedure. **(B)** Recession. The muscle is dissected, disinserted, and then reattached along the path of the inferior oblique muscle but closer to its origin.

An inferior oblique recession acts by inducing muscle slack, thus reducing muscle tension. This is accomplished by moving the muscle insertion closer to the origin, up along the arc of contact of the muscle (Figure 17.2B). Fink described an 8 mm recession site and Apt subsequently found this site by measuring a point 4 mm posterior and 4.4 mm superior to the inferior rectus insertion.[1] Parks suggested placing the muscle close to the vortex vein for moderate inferior oblique overaction.[2] A newer procedure, the anteriorization procedure has improved outcomes, especially for the treatment of severe inferior oblique overaction and is described below. The graded anteriorization procedure is the author's procedure of choice for mild to severe inferior oblique overaction.

## Anteriorization Procedure

The anteriorization procedure changes the vector of forces by moving the inferior oblique muscle insertion anterior towards the inferior rectus insertion (Figure 17.3). This changes the inferior oblique from an elevator to more of a depressor.

### Graded Recession: Anteriorization

The basis of the graded anteriorization procedure is that the more anterior the inferior oblique insertion, the greater the weakening effect (Figure 17.4). This procedure tailors the amount of anteriorization to the amount of inferior oblique overaction. In the mid 1980s, the author developed a modification of the anteriorization procedure based on keeping the posterior fibers behind the inferior rectus insertion, to prevent limitation of elevation, and a graded anterior placement of the muscle depending on the severity of the inferior oblique overaction. This technique, called Graded Anteriorization, was introduced in the first edition of this book (1990). Results of the graded anteriorization have been excellent with over 90% success rate for mild to severe inferior oblique overaction.[3]

Table 17.1 shows the inferior oblique placement for a specific amount of inferior oblique overaction.

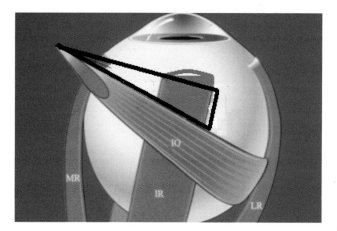

**FIGURE 17.3.** Anteriorization of the inferior oblique muscle consists of moving the insertion to the temporal border of the inferior rectus muscle close to the inferior rectus insertion. Note the anteriorization is shown in black and the new insertion is parallel to the inferior rectus muscle.

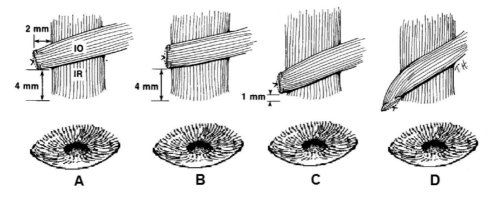

FIGURE 17.4. The diagram shows the "Graded Anteriorization" developed by the author. The more anterior the new insertion the greater the weakening effect. **(A)** This figure shows the least amount of anteriorization for minimal inferior oblique overaction. **(B)** The muscle is placed 4 mm posterior to the inferior rectus insertion for moderate overaction. **(C)** The anteriorization procedure for severe overaction is shown. **(D)** Anteriorization of the entire inferior oblique insertion, including the posterior fibers. Anteriorization of the posterior fibers creates a "J" deformity and limits elevation of the eye.

TABLE 17.1. Management of Inferior Oblique Overaction

| Overaction | Inferior Oblique Placement |
| --- | --- |
| +1 | 4 mm posterior and 2 mm lateral to IR insertion |
| +2 | 3 mm to 4 mm posterior to IR insertion |
| +3 | 1 mm to 2 mm posterior to IR insertion |
| +4 | At IR insertion |
| DVD & IOOA | Full anteriorization with "J" deformity (usually bilateral) |

Although the above table provides guidelines for managing inferior oblique overaction, the final surgical decision must be based on a combination of factors, including the amount of V pattern and the presence of a vertical deviation in primary position. If no vertical deviation is present in primary position, then consider symmetrical surgery. Asymmetric graded anteriorization is indicated if a hypertropia is present. More anteriorization of the inferior oblique should be done on the side of the hypertropia. A full anteriorization (with no "J" deformity) on the side of the hypertropia and 4 mm anteriorization on the opposite side will correct approximately 6 PD of hypertropia. In the case of a unilateral inferior oblique overaction (e.g., associated with congenital superior oblique paresis), an anteriorization with no "J" deformity can correct up to 18 PD of hypertropia. The "J" deformity anteriorization is associated with limited elevation[4] so it is rarely used, except if performed bilaterally for severe DVD and inferior oblique overaction (see "J" Deformity Anteriorization below).

### "J" Deformity Anteriorization

Placement of the posterior fibers at, or anterior to, the inferior rectus insertion produces a "J" deformity, and will limit elevation of the eye (Figure 17.5). The complication of limited elevation has been termed by Mims et al as anti-elevation syndrome.[4] Stager has shown, through anatomical

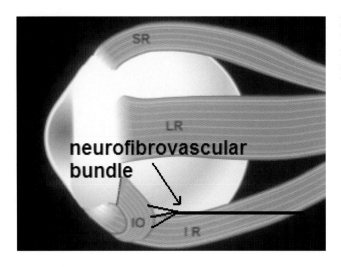

**FIGURE 17.5.** Drawing shows the "J" deformity anteriorization and the neurofibrovascular bundle inserting into the posterior fibers of the inferior oblique muscle. When the posterior muscle fibers are moved anterior to the inferior rectus insertion the neurofibrovascular bundle tethers the eye, resulting in limited elevation.

dissections, that the neurofibrovascular bundle of the inferior oblique inserts into the posterior fibers and can act as a tether to hold the eye down. He found that the ligamentous structure of the neurofibrovascular bundle provides the ancillary origin for the posterior temporal fibers of the inferior oblique muscle when its insertion is transposed anteriorly.[5] Because of these concerns, the full anteriorization with a "J" deformity should be reserved for severe bilateral DVD with inferior oblique overaction. Mims stated that the author's procedure of keeping the posterior fibers posterior to the inferior rectus insertion prevents this complication.

*Effect of Inferior Oblique Weakening on Horizontal Deviation*

If inferior oblique overaction is associated with horizontal strabismus, surgery for inferior oblique dysfunction should be performed along with the horizontal strabismus surgery. Weakening the inferior oblique muscle will not significantly alter the horizontal alignment in primary position. When planning simultaneous horizontal and inferior oblique surgery, the amount of horizontal surgery should be based on the measurement in primary position, independent of the inferior oblique surgery.

## Surgical Technique

An important anatomic consideration in choosing the correct surgical technique is the proximity of the inferior oblique muscle insertion to the macula. A misadventure with a stray needle in this area can cause loss of central vision. We now use the Wright grooved hook to protect the macula during needle passes through the muscle insertion. Another consideration is the course of the inferior temporal vortex vein, which lies underneath the inferior oblique and can be inadvertently traumatized during surgery. Extraconal fat around the inferior oblique muscle is also an important concern. Violating Tenon's capsule in this area can cause the fat adherence syndrome and postoperative restriction. A head lamp is suggested for locating the inferior oblique muscle, because it is located in a "hole" underneath the lower lid, and is not illuminated well with overhead lighting.

The technique described below is a left inferior oblique muscle recession with anteriorization 4 mm posterior to the inferior rectus insertion. The technique for securing the inferior oblique muscle can be used for a variety of procedures including recession, myectomy and extirpation/denervation. The placement of the inferior oblique insertion for a graded anteriorization is described in Figure 17.4. A description of inferior oblique myectomy and extirpation/denervation of the inferior oblique appears later in this chapter.

*Inferior Oblique Anteriorization Left Eye*

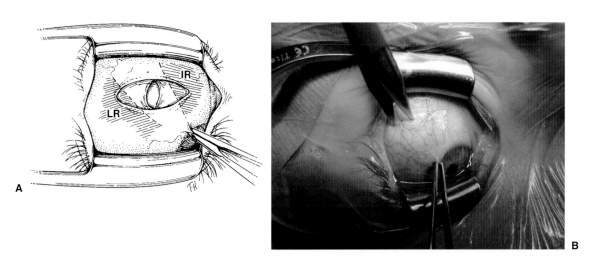

**FIGURE 17.6. (A)** The conjunctival incision parallel to the lid speculum and the deeper intermuscular septum incision perpendicular to the conjunctival incision. The incision is located between the inferior and lateral rectus muscles. **(B)** The conjunctival incision being made parallel to the lid speculum with the blunt Westcott scissors. Make the incision 2 mm to 3 mm anterior to the extraconal fat pad.

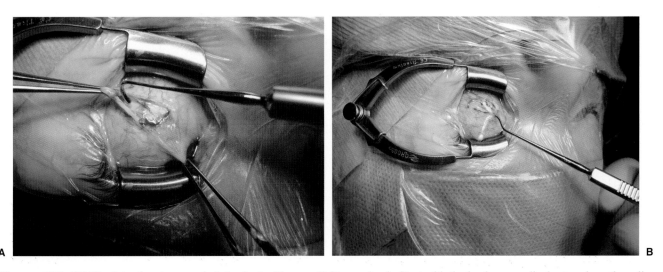

**FIGURE 17.7. (A)** The lateral rectus muscle is hooked with a small Stevens hook. Start with the hook perpendicular to sclera, then slip the hook posterior behind the lateral rectus muscle. **(B)** Replace the Stevens hook with a large Jameson hook. Use the Jameson hook to pull the eye up and in (nasally) to expose the inferior temporal quadrant. The photograph shows the Jameson hook behind the lateral rectus muscle pulling the eye up and in. Note that the cornea is not seen in the photograph, as it is buried in the superior nasal quadrant to expose the inferior temporal quadrant.

## Traction Suture Option

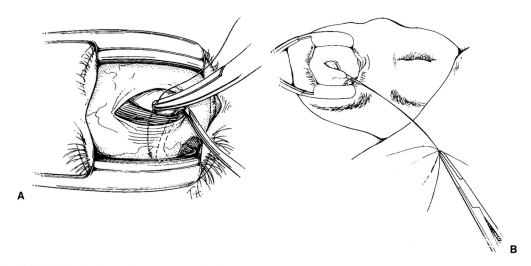

**FIGURE 17.8.** (**A**) A 4-0 black silk traction suture is placed behind the lateral rectus muscle. (**B**) The traction suture pulls the eye up and in to expose the inferior temporal quadrant. To expose the posterior border of the inferior oblique muscle, rotate the eye to an extreme superior nasal position. The traction suture is clamped to the head drape.

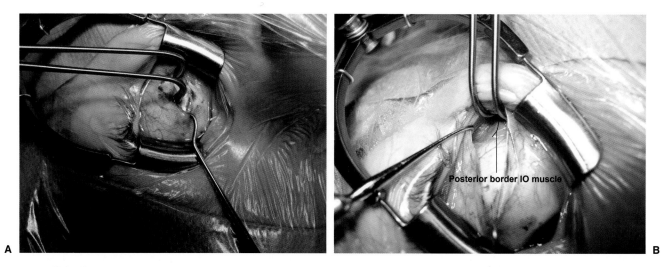

**FIGURE 17.9.** (**A**) A Wright double hook is placed in the inferior temporal quadrant to expose the inferior oblique muscle. The Wright double hook is made of titanium, and consists of two large smooth hooks mounted on a single handle. It is designed to flex so it moulds to the opening in the conjunctiva, enhancing the exposure of the inferior oblique muscle with a single hook. An alternative is to use one or two von Graefe hooks, as shown in Figure 17.10 and 17.11. (**B**) The inferior oblique muscle and the posterior border are shown. The key to hooking the entire inferior oblique muscle is visualizing the posterior border of the muscle.

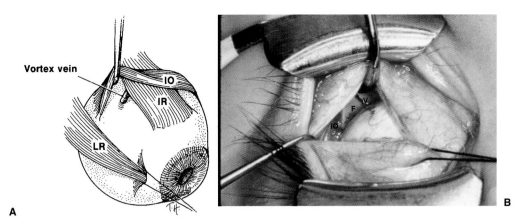

**FIGURE 17.10.** **(A)** The anatomical relationship among the inferior oblique muscle, lateral rectus muscle, inferior rectus muscle, and the vortex vein. Note that the vortex vein is close to the posterior border of the inferior oblique muscle, and can be inadvertently ruptured during hooking the muscle. **(B)** The inferior oblique muscle is exposed. A small Stevens hook is placed along the inferior border of the lateral rectus muscle, and a large von Graefe hook is placed posteriorly under the inferior oblique muscle. Raising the hook (Wright or von Graefe) allows visualization of the area between the inferior oblique and sclera. The following structures are labeled; inferior oblique muscle (IO), orbital fat behind Tenon's capsule (F), and vortex vein (V). A head lamp should be used to illuminate this area.

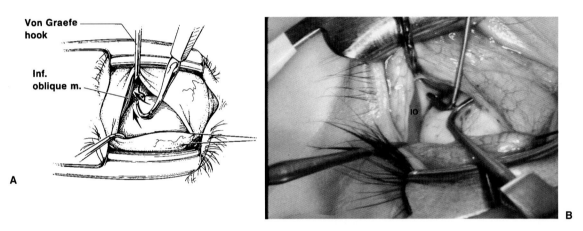

**FIGURE 17.11.** **(A)** Once the posterior border of the inferior oblique is identified by direct visualization, a Stevens hook is placed just behind the posterior border and rotated to hook the entire muscle. The muscle is delivered into the surgical field, keeping the tip of the Stevens hook up and the end of the hook down, to prevent the muscle from slipping off the tip of the hook. Muscle slippage can split a muscle, a common cause of missed fibers and residual inferior oblique overaction. **(B)** The Stevens hook at the posterior border of the inferior oblique muscle is shown. Notice a second small hook gently depresses sclera to expose the posterior anatomy.

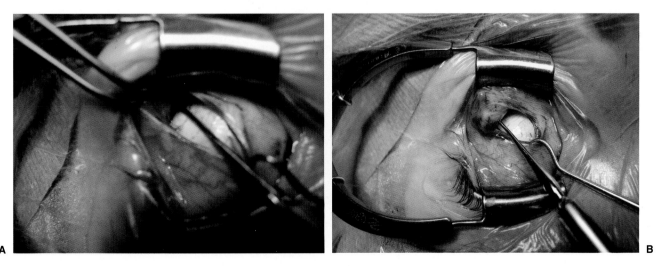

**FIGURE 17.12.** **(A)** The inferior oblique muscle is hooked and gently pulled into the surgical field. **(B)** Tenon's capsule, intermuscular septum and encapsulated fat are also hooked and surround the inferior oblique muscle.

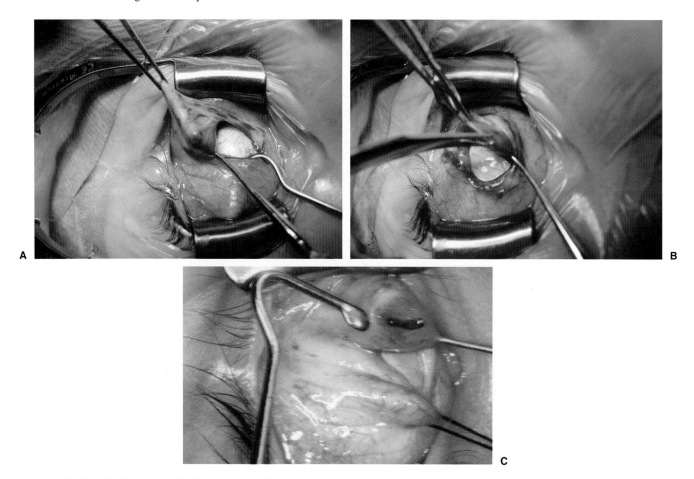

**FIGURE 17.13.** **(A)** The tissues that have been inadvertently hooked are removed by gently lifting the tissues up and off the end of the Stevens hook with a 2 × 3 Lester forceps. Drop the tip of the Stevens hook slightly while the forceps pull the fascial tissue off the hook. **(B)** After removing perimuscular fascial tissue, the intermuscular septum is pulled over the tip of the Stevens hook with the 2 × 3 Lester forceps. Intermuscular septum is opened with the Westcott scissors cutting close to the tip of the muscle hook. This bares the tip of Stevens hook and exposes the edge of the inferior oblique muscle. Do not make cuts deep in the fornix, as this will violate the posterior Tenon's capsule, causing fat adherence and postoperative restriction. **(C)** The Stevens hook is shown around the inferior oblique muscle after intermuscular septum has been removed. A Jameson hook is passed through the hole in the intermuscular septum and behind the inferior oblique muscle.

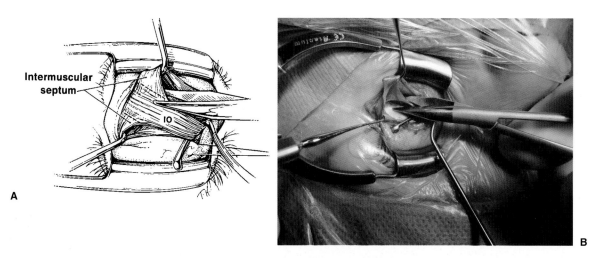

**FIGURE 17.14.** **(A)** Two Stevens hooks are placed above and below the inferior oblique muscle to expose and stretch intermuscular septum. The inferior oblique is pulled nasally by the Jameson hook as the two Stevens hooks pull up laterally. A careful dissection toward the inferior oblique insertion is performed. Dissect close to the muscle belly to remove intermuscular septum from above and below the inferior oblique muscle. The ligament between the lateral rectus and inferior oblique should also be removed. **(B)** Blunt Westcott scissors dissecting intermuscular septum from inferior oblique muscle, keeping close to the muscle, and avoiding the posterior Tenon's capsule and fat. Check ligaments to the inferior oblique are best removed by a combination of blunt and sharp dissection.

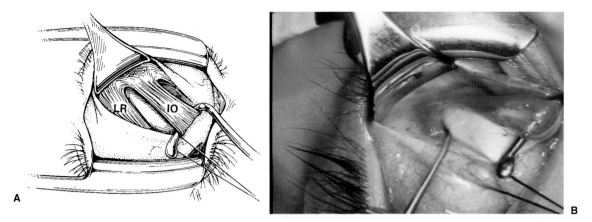

**FIGURE 17.15. (A)** At this point, the inferior oblique muscle is clearly exposed and isolated for any desired procedure. Notice that the lateral rectus is just superior to the inferior oblique muscle. **(B)** The photograph shows the inferior oblique muscle clear of intermuscular septum. The lateral rectus muscle is being pulled superiorly with the Stevens hook, and the other Stevens hook has been replaced by a medium-sized Desmarres retractor. Most of the ligament between the inferior oblique and lateral rectus has been dissected.

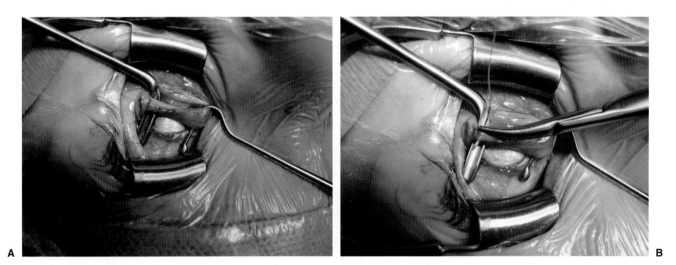

**FIGURE 17.16. (A)** The Wright grooved hook is placed under the inferior oblique and pulled temporally toward the insertion. The Jameson hook is pulled in the opposite direction (nasally) so the Wright grooved hook can be placed firmly against the inferior oblique insertion. **(B)** The needle is being passed through the inferior oblique muscle insertion, approximately 3 mm from the sclera, over the Wright grooved hook. Wright grooved hook protects the sclera against inadvertent scleral perforation. A scleral perforation in this area is especially dangerous, as it will cause a macular tear.

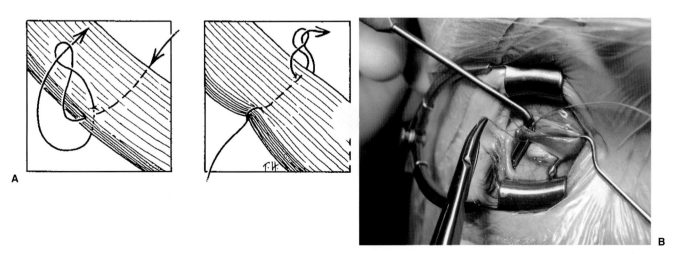

**FIGURE 17.17. (A)** The inferior oblique muscle is secured with a 5-0 Vicryl suture on a spatula needle. The suture is first passed through half thickness of the muscle belly, and locking bites are placed at each edge of the muscle. **(B)** A twist lock keeps the suture from loosening after the muscle is disinserted. **OPTION:** An alternative technique is to disinsert the muscle first and then pass the needles and secure the muscle away from the globe.

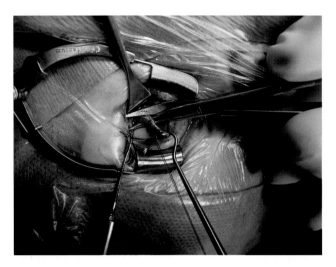

**FIGURE 17.18.** The inferior oblique muscle has been secured with a double-arm suture and is being disinserted with the blunt Westcott scissors. Do not cut too close to the sclera. A cut suture is not a major problem because you will never lose an inferior oblique muscle, but stay away from the sclera because the inferior oblique inserts near the macula. Removing the inferior oblique at its insertion does not cause significant bleeding, and routine clamping of the muscle is not necessary. After the inferior oblique muscle is disinserted, remove the 4-0 silk traction suture that is behind the lateral rectus muscle.

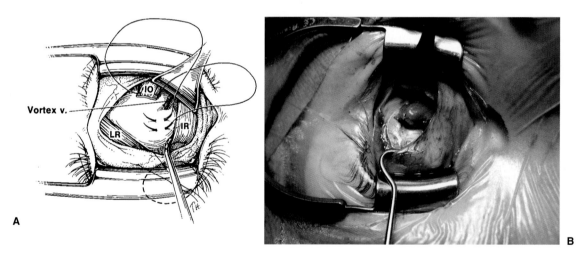

**FIGURE 17.19.** (**A**) The muscle is reattached to the globe at the desired anteriorization point. In this case, the muscle is being placed along the temporal border of the inferior rectus muscle 4mm posterior to its insertion. A Desmarres retractor is positioned to retract the conjunctiva and Tenon's capsule. Note that the needles are placed along the temporal border of the inferior rectus muscle, with the posterior suture placed behind the anterior suture. (**B**) The inferior oblique muscle tied in place along the temporal border of the inferior rectus muscle. The intermuscular septum and conjunctiva are closed separately with 6-0 plain gut suture.

## Myectomy

The inferior oblique muscle is isolated and exposed, as described earlier in this chapter.

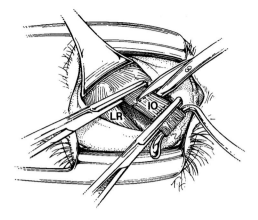

FIGURE 17.20.  The entire width of the inferior oblique muscle is cross-clamped with two small hemostats. The hemostats should be placed approximately 8 mm apart, with one near the inferior oblique insertion, and the other near the temporal border of the inferior rectus muscle. The muscle between the clamps is then excised with the West-cott scissors, cutting close to the hemostats. Cautery is applied to the muscle stumps, and the hemostats are removed.

## Extirpation/Denervation of the Inferior Oblique Muscle

The extirpation/denervation procedure should be performed only on extremely overacting inferior oblique muscles, or when a previous myectomy or anteriorization procedure has failed. The author rarely uses this procedure.

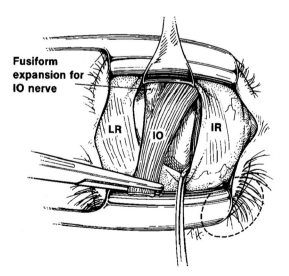

FIGURE 17.21.  The inferior oblique has been isolated and detached from the globe by the standard fornix incision technique. Westcott scissors are used to dissect along the inferior oblique muscle toward its origin. The inferior oblique muscle is pulled superolaterally, to identify a fusiform expansion on the posterior border. This fusiform expansion represents the insertion of the neurofibrovascular bundle into the inferior oblique muscle.

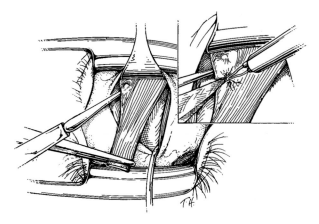

**FIGURE 17.22.** The nerve and vessels are hooked with a small Stevens hook, and tension on the Stevens hook identifies a tight band. Cautery is used to cut through this tight band. Once the nerve has been severed, the inferior oblique will release, confirming that the nerve has been cut. The inset provides a magnified view of the cautery used to cut the inferior oblique nerve and companion vessel. Place a sponge under the muscle to protect the sclera from the cautery.

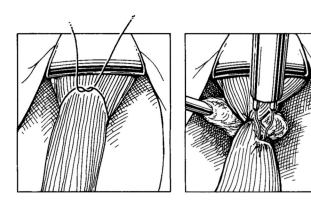

**FIGURE 17.23.** A 4-0 Vicryl suture is placed around the entire inferior oblique muscle close to its origin, and tied tightly. A cotton-tip applicator is placed underneath the muscle, and distal muscle is removed by cauterizing through the muscle. After the muscle is removed, the surrounding Tenon's capsule is sutured over the muscle stump with 7-0 Vicryl to internalize the stump.

## Complications

The most common complication of inferior oblique surgery is persistence or recurrence of the overaction. A common cause of residual overaction is incomplete isolation of the inferior oblique muscle, leaving posterior fibers intact. It is important to explore posteriorly along the globe, for bridging muscle fibers that indicate missed inferior oblique muscle fibers.

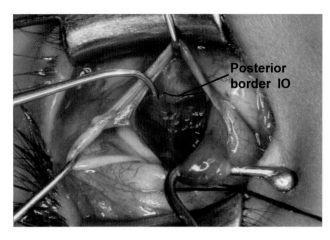

FIGURE 17.24. This is an example of a split left inferior oblique muscle with missed posterior muscle fibers. The eye is rotated up and in by a black silk traction suture, which encircles the lateral rectus muscle. The large Jameson hook in the foreground has hooked part of the inferior oblique muscle and is pulling it superiorly. Residual inferior oblique muscle is seen deep in the fornix, and a small Stevens hook is being placed behind the missed fibers.

Fat adherence syndrome is another important complication. It occurs most often when the inferior oblique muscle is hooked blindly and posterior Tenon's capsule is violated. Dr. Marshall Parks first discovered the fat adherence syndrome in a patient who had undergone inferior oblique surgery. Other possible complications of inferior oblique surgery include anterior orbital hemorrhage, pupillary dilation, damage or inadvertent surgery to the lateral rectus muscle, and even visual loss caused by ocular penetration in the macular area. Paramount in avoiding these complications is the clear and direct visualization of the inferior oblique muscle during its isolation. Blind hooking procedures must be avoided. Meticulous surgical dissection and hemostasis are the key to proper exposure and visualization of the anatomy.

Weakening procedures of the inferior oblique muscle for primary congenital overaction only rarely produce a postoperative torsional diplopia. Even so, an adult patient may complain of a transient excyclodiplopia after weakening of the inferior oblique muscle.

## References

1. Apt L, Call NB. Inferior oblique muscle recession. Am J Ophthalmol 1978;85:95–100.
2. Parks MM, Inferior oblique weakening procedures. Int Ophthalmol Clin 1985;25:107–117.
3. Guemes A, Wright KW. Effect of graded anterior transposition of the inferior oblique muscle on versions and vertical deviation in primary position. J AAPOS 1998;2:201–206.
4. Mims JL, Wood RC. Antielevation syndrome after bilateral anterior transposition of the inferior oblique muscles: incidence and prevention. J AAPOS 1999;3:333–336.
5. Stager DR, Costenbader lecture. Anatomy and surgery of the inferior oblique muscle: recent findings. J AAPOS 2001;5:203–208.

# 18 Superior Oblique Tendon Tightening Procedures

## Physiology of Superior Oblique Tendon Tightening Procedures

The superior oblique tendon can be functionally divided into the anterior third, which is responsible for intorsion, and the posterior two-thirds, which is responsible for depression and abduction (Figure 18.1). Superior oblique tightening procedures are based on this physiologic division and either tighten the whole tendon (i.e., full tendon tuck) or tighten the anterior tendon fibers (i.e., the Harada-Ito procedure).

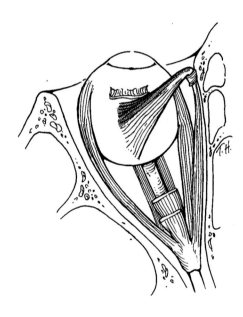

FIGURE 18.1. The anterior fibers of the left superior oblique tendon are shaded. These fibers course close to the equator of the eye and are responsible for intorsion. Posterior fibers are behind the equator and lift the back of the eye toward the trochlea, effecting abduction and depression.

### *Full Tendon Tuck*

A full tendon tuck tightens both anterior and posterior fibers, and enhances all three functions of the superior oblique muscle. This operation is useful for correcting extorsion, hyperdeviation that increases in the field of action of the superior oblique, and convergence in down gaze. Tightening of the entire superior oblique tendon can, however, lead to limited elevation in adduction or an iatrogenic Brown's syndrome. Care must be taken to balance the superior oblique tightening against an induced Brown's syndrome, by performing intraoperative forced ductions of the superior oblique tendon after tucking.

*Harada-Ito Procedure*

There are clinical circumstances that require selective correction of extorsion without a significant change in vertical or horizontal alignment. A full tendon tuck in this situation is not appropriate because it would induce a hypotropia, and possibly cause an iatrogenic Brown's syndrome. The Harada-Ito procedure is designed to selectively correct extorsion by tightening only the anterior superior oblique fibers. The "Harada-Ito plus" procedure incorporates a few millimeters of the more posterior tendon, and improves posterior tendon function. This procedure can correct small hypertropias in addition to extorsion.

## Isolation and Exposure of the Superior Oblique Tendon (Left Eye: Surgeon's View)

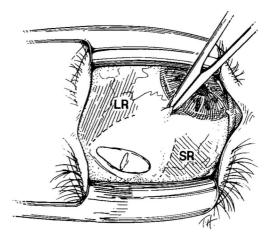

**FIGURE 18.2.** With the eye depressed and adducted by the assistant, a superior temporal fornix incision is made approximately 8 mm posterior to the limbus as described in Chapter 11.

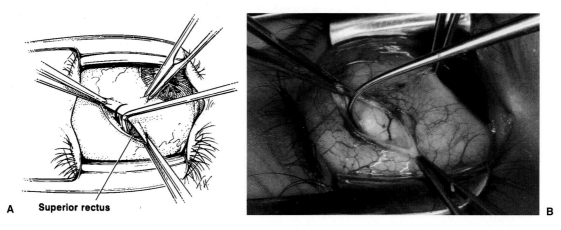

**A   Superior rectus**

**B**

**FIGURE 18.3. (A)** The temporal border of the superior rectus muscle is identified visually and hooked at the insertion, first with the small Stevens hook, and then with the larger Green or Jameson hook. Do not sweep posteriorly when hooking the superior rectus muscle or the anterior fibers of the superior oblique tendon insertion will be inadvertently hooked, or even disinserted. The idea is to preserve the integrity of the entire superior oblique insertion. **(B)** The Stevens hook on bare sclera ready to hook the lateral pole of the left superior rectus muscle insertion. A small triangle of the right superior rectus muscle is seen between the tip of the hook and the forceps to the right.

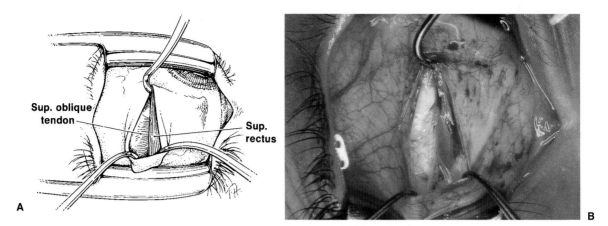

**FIGURE 18.4. (A)** Using the Jameson hook to retract the superior rectus, the globe is maximally depressed, and the incision is opened with two small hooks to expose the temporal border of the superior rectus muscle. A limited dissection of check ligaments overlying the temporal third of the superior rectus muscle may be necessary to gain posterior exposure. Stay on top of the muscle, being careful not to dissect fascial tissue off the temporal sclera. **(B)** The temporal border of the superior rectus muscle with a large hook retracting the superior rectus muscle to rotate the globe inferiorly. The temporal border of the superior rectus muscle can be seen. The fine tissue overlying the sclera just temporal to the superior rectus muscle represents the fanned out portion of the superior oblique tendon covered with a thin layer of intermuscular septum. Do not clean the temporal aspect of the superior rectus muscle and do not excise the temporal intermuscular septum. Because it is closely adherent to the fanned out portion of the superior oblique tendon, removing the intermuscular septum in this area often inadvertently removes the superior oblique tendon.

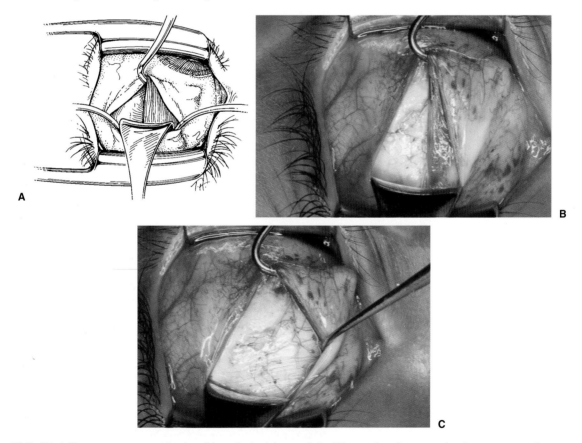

**FIGURE 18.5. (A)** A Desmarres retractor is placed into the incision, and the lid speculum is removed to improve posterior exposure. **(B)** The photograph shows the temporal border of the superior rectus muscle and superior oblique tendon covered with intermuscular septum. Note that it is difficult to visualize the fibers of the superior oblique insertion, and the tissue temporal to the superior rectus muscle can be easily mistaken for intermuscular septum. **(C)** A small hook is placed underneath the belly of the superior rectus muscle and is retracted nasally to expose the fibers of the superior oblique tendon. The superior oblique tendon fibers are identified by their parallel pattern and their white, glistening appearance. These fibers run under and perpendicular to the fibers of the superior rectus muscle.

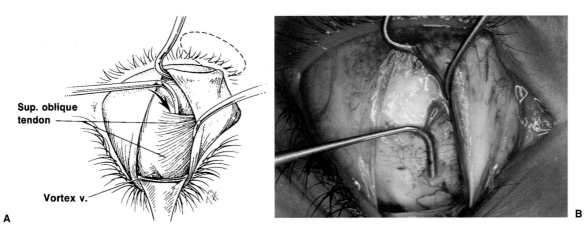

**FIGURE 18.6. (A)** The anterior fibers of the superior oblique tendon are hooked with a small Stevens hook along the temporal border of the superior rectus muscle. The tendon is exposed and ready for surgical manipulation. **(B)** A small Stevens hook is shown behind the anterior fibers and superior oblique tendon. The vortex vein can be seen as a purple coloration in the sclera, just under the Desmarres retractor, at the most posterior aspect of the incision.

## Harada-Ito Procedure

The Harada-Ito procedure tightens the anterior superior oblique tendon fibers, thus inducing intorsion without significantly affecting the posterior tendon functions of abduction and depression. Described below are two techniques for tightening the anterior fibers: disinsertion technique and classic Harada-Ito procedure.

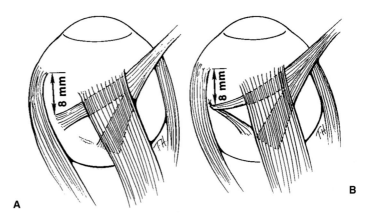

**FIGURE 18.7. (A)** With the disinsertion technique, the anterior fibers of the superior oblique tendon are sutured, then disinserted and moved anteriorly and laterally, to be secured to sclera at a point 8 mm posterior to the superior border of the lateral rectus insertion. Lateralizing the anterior fibers intorts the eye, thus correcting extorsion. **(B)** In the classic Harada-Ito procedure, the anterior superior oblique tendon fibers are looped with a suture and displaced laterally without disinsertion. The anterior superior oblique tendon fibers are sutured to sclera 8 mm posterior to the superior border of the lateral rectus muscle.

## Disinsertion Harada-Ito Technique

Exposure and isolation of the anterior fibers of the superior oblique tendon are performed through a superior temporal fornix incision as described previously (Figures 18.2 to 18.6).

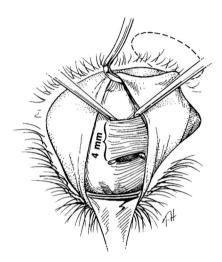

**FIGURE 18.8.** The anterior fibers of the superior oblique tendon are isolated with two small muscle hooks, and the tendon is divided by separating the two hooks by approximately 6 mm to 8 mm apart. Only the anterior quarter of the tendon (approximately 4 mm of tendon) is isolated.

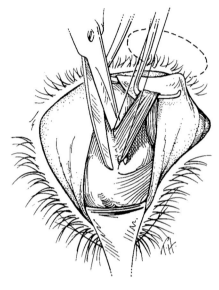

**FIGURE 18.9.** The anterior superior oblique tendon fibers are secured with a 5-0 Mersilene double arm suture (nonabsorbable suture) with spatula needles. Locking bites are placed at each edge of the isolated anterior tendon fibers. The anterior tendon fibers are disinserted, with the Westcott scissors, close to the sclera.

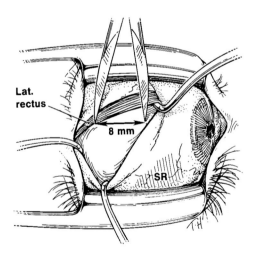

**FIGURE 18.10.** The superior rectus muscle is released, and a large hook is placed behind the lateral rectus muscle, pulling the eye into adduction. Calipers are used to measure 8 mm posterior to the superior pole of the lateral rectus muscle, where the anterior half of the tendon will be sutured to the sclera. Place the anterior fibers 8 mm posterior to the lateral rectus insertion to avoid anteriorizing the superior oblique fibers, and possibly creating a consecutive esodeviation.

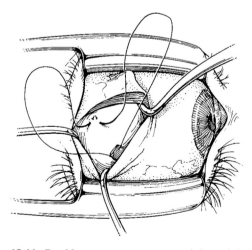

**FIGURE 18.11.** Double arm sutures are passed through half thickness sclera at the superior border of the lateral rectus muscle, 8 mm posterior to the superior pole of the lateral rectus muscle insertion. The needles exit close together, nearly touching each other.

**FIGURE 18.12.** The needles are withdrawn from the sclera, and the sutures are pulled to advance the anterior tendon laterally, while the eye is intorted by rotating it with the large hook. The tendon should be pulled tight and the sutures tied together. If intraoperative adjustment of torsion based on indirect ophthalmoscopy is going to be performed, then tie a bow-tie knot to temporarily secure the tendon.

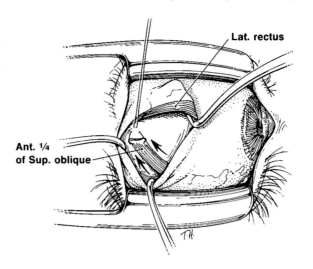

*Intraoperative Adjustment of Torsion (Guyton Technique)*

Intraoperative torsional adjustment can be made by comparing objective retinal torsion before and after the Harada-Ito procedure. Adjustment is made by first observing the torsional position of the fundus with the indirect ophthalmoscope before the anterior superior oblique tendon fibers are tightened. Note the position of the fovea in relationship to the optic disc. In a normal eye, a horizontal line drawn from the fovea should intersect the inferior half of the disc (upper half of the disc, as seen through the indirect view). Next, tighten the anterior fibers to induce intorsion, and tie the anterior fibers in place with a bow-tie. Reexamine the fundus with the indirect ophthalmoscope noting the change in the foveal position. Because the indirect view is inverted, induced intorsion will produce an apparent inferior shift in the position of the fovea relative to the optic disc. A shift of 1/2 disc diameter will produce approximately 10° of intorsional change. If after tightening the anterior superior oblique tendon fibers, the objective torsional change is not satisfactory, the lateral rectus is again hooked, and the anterior fibers are either tightened or loosened to obtain the desired result. It is more important to monitor the net change in foveal position than to emphasize the exact position of the fovea, as the foveal position will undoubtedly change when the patient is awake and not under the influence of anesthesia. Once the desired amount of intorsional change is achieved, the bow-tie is cut and the knot is tied in a permanent fashion. This technique can be used with both the disinsertion and classical Harada-Ito procedure.

*Adjustable Suture Technique*

The Harada-Ito procedure can be transformed into an adjustable suture technique by placing a noose around the sutures as they exit sclera. The noose mechanics are identical to the standard rectus adjustable suture technique. The endpoint for adjustment is elimination of torsional diplopia, with special attention to correcting the extorsion in down gaze. The anterior fibers can be advanced or released to achieve the desired result. The adjustment can be difficult for the patient and it is often hard to titrate the adjustment endpoint, so this author has all but abandoned the adjustable Harada-Ito procedure. Results with the fixed suture classic Harada-Ito procedure have been excellent.

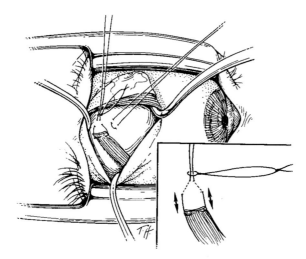

**FIGURE 18.13.** The diagram shows the adjustable suture apparatus with a noose placed around exiting scleral sutures. Notice that a traction suture is placed a few millimeters anterior to the adjustable suture apparatus and is secured to sclera. The traction suture helps to retract the conjunctiva at the time of adjustment and manipulates the eye position to gain posterior exposure.

## Classic Harada-Ito Technique

This procedure has the advantage of being easily reversible, and is the technique of choice for the author. To undo the classic Harada-Ito, simply cut the suture and the tendon will be back to normal. This must be done within 24 to 48 hours after surgery or the tendon will scar in place. The following instructions assume that the left superior oblique tendon has been identified, and that the anterior quarter of the superior oblique tendon has been identified and separated (see the description earlier in this chapter).

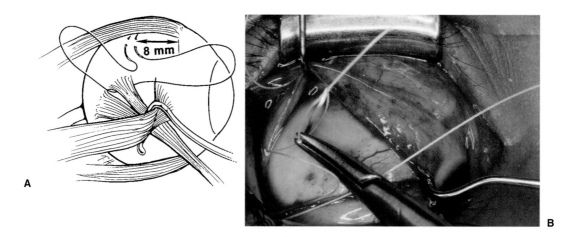

**FIGURE 18.14. (A)** A 5-0 Mersilene double arm suture with spatula needles is passed behind the anterior one-quarter (approximately 4 mm) of the superior oblique tendon. The anterior fibers are separated from the posterior fibers for 6 mm to 8 mm from the insertion. This suture passes beneath, not through, the anterior tendon. Both needles are then passed at the superior border of the lateral rectus muscle, 8 mm posterior to the lateral rectus insertion, in a parallel fashion, exiting close together. **(B)** The needle is passed toward the lateral rectus muscle, 8 mm posterior to the lateral rectus insertion. The large hook is behind the lateral rectus muscle, and pulls the eye into adduction. It is important to place the sutures 8 mm posterior to the lateral rectus insertion, as anterior placement of the superior oblique tendon fibers can induce an esodeviation.

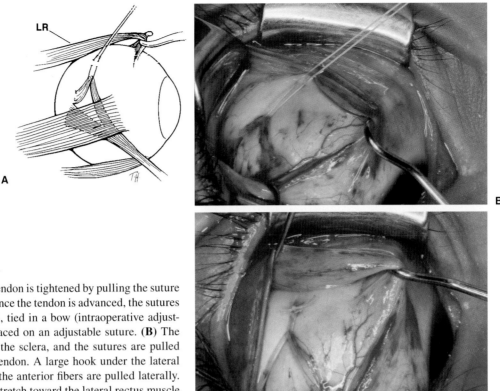

**FIGURE 18.15.** **(A)** The anterior tendon is tightened by pulling the suture toward the lateral rectus muscle. Once the tendon is advanced, the sutures can be tied in place (fixed suture), tied in a bow (intraoperative adjustment of torsion; see above), or placed on an adjustable suture. **(B)** The needles have been removed from the sclera, and the sutures are pulled laterally to advance the anterior tendon. A large hook under the lateral rectus is used to intort the eye as the anterior fibers are pulled laterally. **(C)** The anterior fibers placed on stretch toward the lateral rectus muscle with scleral sutures tied off. Notice the large hook is placed behind the lateral rectus muscle.

## Full Tendon Superior Oblique Tuck

### Technique Using Greene Tendon Tucker

The temporal fibers of the left superior rectus are isolated through a superior temporal fornix incision (see Figures 18.2 to 18.6). A large hook behind the superior rectus muscle depresses the eye while a Desmarres retractor retracts the conjunctiva to gain posterior exposure.

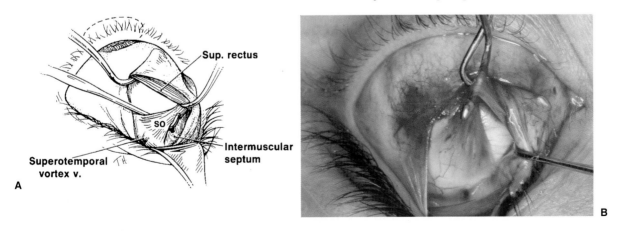

**FIGURE 18.16.** **(A)** The lid speculum has been removed. A Stevens hook is passed beneath the superior oblique tendon until the posterior border can be identified by direct visualization and the full, fanned out insertion of the tendon is on the muscle hook. Because the superior temporal vortex vein usually penetrates the sclera near the junction of the posterior one-third and anterior two-thirds of the tendon insertion, it is advisable to visually identify this vein before hooking the posterior aspect of the tendon to avoid rupture. The intermuscular septum is incised anteriorly and posteriorly, clearing the distal portion of the tendon for tucking. **(B)** The superior oblique insertion with the tendon on a Jameson hook. The broad fanned tendon has been cleared of the intermuscular septum. The superior temporal vortex vein is barely seen under the Desmarres retractor.

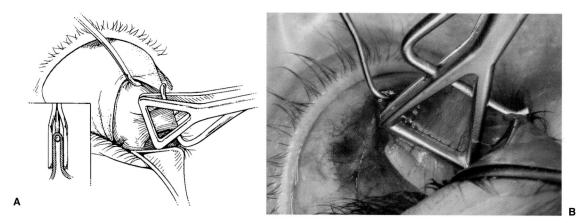

**FIGURE 18.17.** **(A)** The muscle hook holding the superior oblique tendon is replaced with the tendon tucker, which is tightened to take up the slack in the tendon for tucking. *Inset* shows the side view of tendon folded over the large hook inside the tucker. The hook pulls the tendon into the tucker. Many tendon tuckers are available for this purpose; the Greene tucker is illustrated here. The total amount of tuck varies from 6 mm to 15 mm, depending on the degree of tendon laxity. The correct amount of tuck is verified by forced duction testing. **(B)** A temporal view of the superior oblique tendon folded in the tucker. The hook in the tucker is retracted, pulling the tendon into the jaws of the tucker.

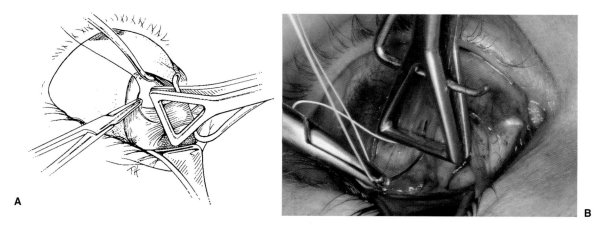

**FIGURE 18.18.** **(A)** The folded tendon is tied together with a 5-0 Mersilene double arm suture passed in a double-mattress fashion. First, the needles are passed through the center of the folded tendon, close to sclera, in the temporal to nasal direction. **(B)** A second needle is being passed under the tucker in a temporal to nasal direction to bind the fibers of the tucked portion of the tendon together.

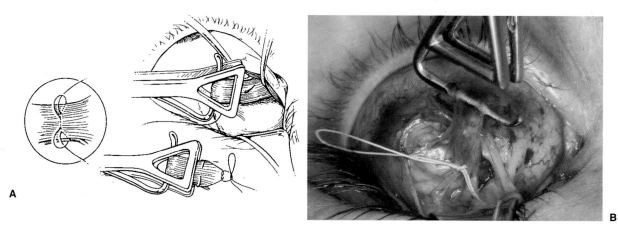

**FIGURE 18.19.** **(A)** The needle exits on the nasal side of folded tendon below the clamp of the Greene tucker. The circle shows the nasal side of tucked tendon with the suture path. There is a central mattress suture linked to two locking bites at each edge of the tendon. The bottom drawing shows the ends of the double arm suture tied together in a single loop bow-tie. **(B)** The folded tendon is tied together close to the scleral insertion with a single loop bow knot. This figure shows the knot on the temporal side of the tendon. The hook inside the tendon tucker clamp is lowered to release the tucked tendon.

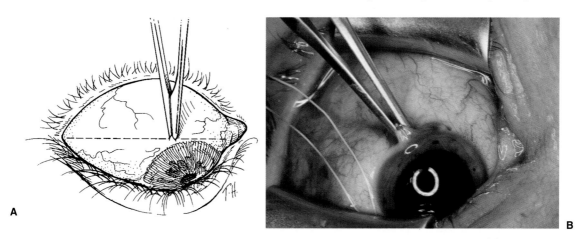

A

B

FIGURE 18.20. **(A)** Forced duction testing is carried out by grasping the globe at the limbus in the inferotemporal quadrant (7:30 o'clock position) and gently moving the eye into elevation and adduction. Resistance, caused by tightening of the superior oblique tendon, should be felt as the inferior limbus reaches an imaginary line drawn between the medial and lateral canthus. If significant resistance is encountered while the inferior limbus is inferior to this line, the tuck is too tight, and a significant iatrogenic Brown's syndrome will result. If resistance is not felt until the inferior limbus is above this imaginary line, the tuck is not tight enough and inadequate correction will occur. It is important to maintain the globe in its proper anterior/posterior position while performing this forced duction test. Do not depress or proptose the globe because the forced duction testing will be inaccurate. **(B)** The figure shows forced ductions up and in, to detect a Brown's syndrome. The inferior limbus is at the point where a significant resistance should be felt. The white suture is the 5-0 Mersilene from the bow-tie on the tucked tendon. If the amount of tuck is too much, as determined by the forced duction test, the temporary Mersilene slip knot is loosened. The tucker can be readjusted for a larger or smaller tuck, and the Mersilene suture is replaced, as previously described.

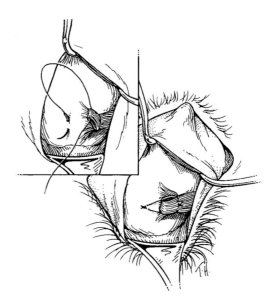

FIGURE 18.21. After the forced duction testing verifies the correct degree of superior oblique tucking, the large muscle hook is placed beneath the superior rectus to depress the globe, and the Desmarres retractor is reinserted to expose the tucked tendon. The Mersilene suture, previously tied in a bow, is permanently tied. A good method is to cut the single bow and remove the extra suture from the knot. This leaves a tied square knot without having to undo the bow, avoiding suture slippage. The diagram shows the tucked tendon with a redundant fold of tendon. *Top left* shows one end of the previously removed Mersilene suture being passed through the tendon temporally, along the line of tendon action, as illustrated *right bottom*. Tacking redundant tendon to sclera is optional and may not be necessary for small tucks.

## Superior Oblique Tendon Plication

*Technique Without Using a Tucker*

The left superior oblique has been isolated and hooked (see the description earlier in this chapter).

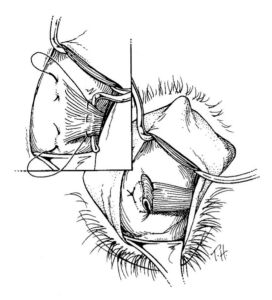

**FIGURE 18.22.** (*Upper left*) The entire width of the superior oblique tendon is hooked (Jameson hook) along the temporal border of the superior rectus muscle. The tendon is secured with a 5-0 Mersilene double arm suture with spatula needles at the desired tuck location, usually 8 mm to 10 mm proximal to the insertion. The first pass is a small, full thickness bite at the center of the tendon, and the sutures are tied together in a square knot (central knot). Each end of the double arm suture is passed behind the tendon, starting at the center and exiting at the tendon edge. Locking bites are placed at each edge of the tendon, and the needles are passed just lateral to the anterior and posterior insertion of the superior oblique tendon with partial thickness scleral bites. (*Lower right*) The needles are withdrawn from the sclera, and the sutures are pulled to tuck the tendon. The sutures are tied together in a bow, and forced ductions are performed to evaluate for a possible Brown's syndrome (see Figure 18.21). The sutures are tied together to secure the tuck. The redundant fold of tendon can be tacked down, but this is optional.

# 19  Superior Oblique Tendon Weakening Procedures

Superior oblique tendon weakening procedures are used in the management of various types of strabismus including superior oblique overaction, inferior oblique palsy, and Brown's syndrome (see Chapter 7). Most procedures weaken the superior oblique muscle by slackening the tendon. Uncontrolled procedures include tenotomy and tenectomy, as the tendon is cut and the cut ends are free to widely separate or scar back together. These uncontrolled procedures should not be used in patients with binocular fusion, as the incidence of consecutive superior oblique palsy is more than 50%.

Controlled lengthening of the tendon grades the induced slack. The two most effective controlled lengthening procedures are the Wright silicone tendon expander and the split tendon elongation procedure. These procedures have significantly reduced the complication of consecutive superior oblique palsy and have had excellent outcomes. The superior oblique recession has been described as a controlled weakening procedure, but it has the disadvantage of changing the characteristics of the superior oblique insertion. Normally the superior oblique insertion spans from the superior rectus insertion to 6 mm from the optic nerve. After recessing the superior oblique one creates a new insertion site. The broad insertion is now collapsed and is nasal and anterior to the original insertion. This new insertion position dramatically changes the superior oblique muscle functions, from a depressor and abductor to an elevator and adductor. The complication of limited depression has been well described following the superior oblique recession procedure. Another controlled elongation procedure is the suture bridge or also called the "chicken stitch." A suture is placed between the cut tendon ends to provide a graded separation. The problem with the suture bridge is the suture provides a scaffolding for fibrosis that can reunite the tendon ends. Reuniting of the tendon ends can result in postoperative undercorrection. The superior oblique silicone tendon expander, and the split tendon elongation procedures, keep the tendon ends apart at a fixed distance and are preferred by the author.

Another type of superior oblique weakening procedure is based on selectively removing the posterior tendon fibers (see Figure 19.15). The idea is to reduce the depression and abduction functions, but prevent postoperative extorsion by leaving the anterior fibers intact. The reason there is relatively little effect is because the procedure is performed on the temporal side of the superior rectus muscle. When the temporal fibers are removed from the sclera, they do not retract; rather, they scar down to the sclera under the superior rectus muscle. The posterior tenectomy procedure may be useful for mild superior oblique overaction but a full tendon lengthening procedure is required for more significant overaction and Brown's syndrome.

## Surgical Exposure for Superior Oblique Tendon Weakening

Superior oblique tendon weakening procedures like tenotomy, Wright's silicone tendon expander, and split tendon elongation should be performed nasal to the superior rectus muscle. Temporal tenotomies usually have minimal effect, as the superior oblique tendon is sandwiched between the superior rectus and the sclera. Another disadvantage of the temporal approach is that the tendon is extremely splayed out at its insertion, making it difficult to hook and isolate all of the posterior superior oblique tendon fibers. Finally, the nasal approach leaves the normally broad insertion intact, maintaining its three important functions of abduction, depression, and intorsion.

The preferred procedure for exposure of the tendon, developed by Dr. Marshall Parks, is to perform the superior oblique surgery nasal to the superior rectus muscle through a temporal conjunctival incision. By placing the conjunctival incision temporal to the superior rectus muscle, then reflecting the incision nasally, the surgeon can keep the nasal intermuscular septum intact minimizing scleral-tendon scarring. Additionally, intact nasal intermuscular septum is important to maintain the anatomical relationships of the superior oblique tendon, and helps reduce the incidence of postoperative superior oblique palsy or limited depression.

*Operative Procedure: Temporal Incision–Nasal Tendon Surgery*

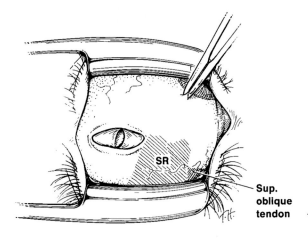

**FIGURE 19.1.** A left eye with a superior temporal fornix incision through conjunctiva, and a separate incision through Tenon's capsule. The conjunctival incision abuts the temporal aspect of the superior rectus muscle.

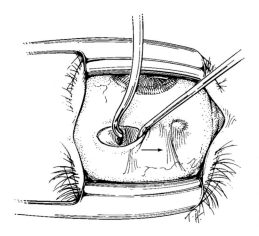

**FIGURE 19.2.** A Jameson hook is placed underneath the superior rectus muscle, and the eye is retracted down. A small Stevens hook is used to pull the incision nasally over the tip of the Jameson hook.

FIGURE 19.3. The conjunctival incision is reflected nasally over the superior rectus insertion. Notice that the bulb tip of the Jameson hook is covered with intermuscular septum. Do not bare the tip of the Jameson hook; instead, leave intermuscular septum intact.

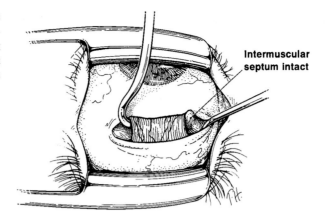

**Intermuscular septum intact**

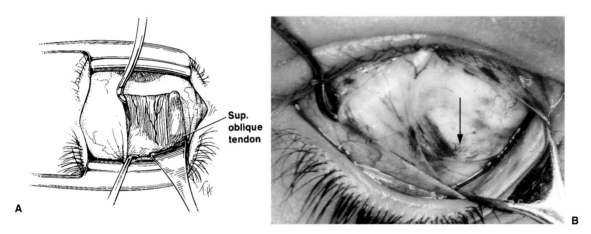

**Sup. oblique tendon**

**A**

**B**

FIGURE 19.4. **(A)** A Desmarres retractor is inserted along the nasal border of the superior rectus muscle, and the lid speculum is removed in order to gain posterior exposure. The superior oblique tendon can be seen, through its fascial covering, as pearly white fibers that run perpendicular to the course of the superior rectus muscle. **(B)** The nasal aspect of the superior rectus muscle is shown. The superior oblique tendon is located nasal to the superior rectus muscle, approximately 12 mm posterior to the superior rectus insertion. Because the superior oblique tendon is surrounded by fascia, it is somewhat difficult to see and is marked by an arrow in the photograph.

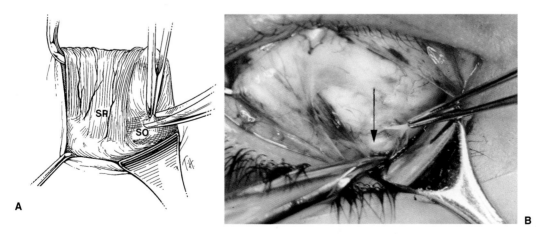

SR  SO

**A**

**B**

FIGURE 19.5. **(A)** A small incision is made over the superior oblique tendon through the fascial covering. This fascial covering is often called the superior oblique sheath or tendon capsule. Keep the nasal intermuscular septum intact by limiting the incision to the width of the tendon. **(B)** Superior oblique tendon fascia has been cut with the Westcott scissors to expose bare tendon. A fine forceps is seen holding the cut edge of the tendon fascia. The pearly white cord to the left of the forceps is the bared superior oblique tendon *(see arrow)*.

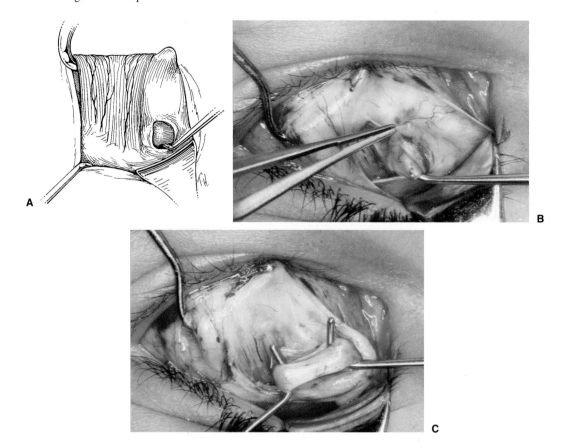

**FIGURE 19.6.** **(A)** The superior oblique tendon is hooked with a small Stevens hook through a small hole in the superior oblique fascia. **(B)** Expose and clear the tendon of fascia by gently lifting the fascial capsule off the tip of the Stevens hook with a 0.3 tooth forceps, as shown here. **(C)** Two small Stevens hooks are spreading the tendon to facilitate the desired surgery: tenotomy, Wright's silicone tendon expander, or split tendon elongation. Note the surrounding tendon capsule and intermuscular septum remains intact.

## Superior Oblique Tenotomy

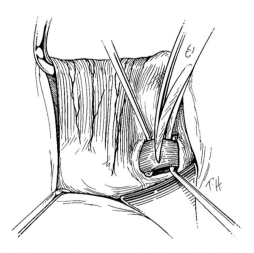

**FIGURE 19.7.** The Westcott scissors are cutting the superior oblique tendon between the two small Stevens hooks. Be sure to perform a complete tenotomy.

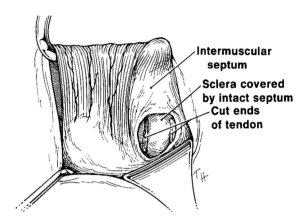

FIGURE 19.8. The cut ends of the superior oblique tendon within the superior oblique fascial compartment are shown. Notice that the fascia surrounding and underlying the superior oblique is intact. After the superior oblique is transected, perform Guyton's exaggerated forced ductions to make sure that the entire tendon has been cut (see Chapter 10). This maneuver is critical because residual tendon yields gross undercorrection. If residual tendon fibers are present, find and cut the fibers.

## Silicone Tendon Expander (Wright Procedure)

### The Superior Oblique Silicone Tendon Expander

This procedure controls the separation of the ends of the tendon, allowing quantification of tendon separation. A segment of a silicone 240 or 40 retinal band is inserted between the cut ends of the superior oblique tendon. The length of silicone is determined by the degree of superior oblique overaction. Remember to take into account the amount of A pattern and downshoot, as observed on versions, when quantitating superior oblique overaction.

| Superior oblique overaction | Length of silicone |
| --- | --- |
| +1 | 4 mm |
| +2 | 5 mm |
| +3 | 6 mm |
| +4 | 7 mm (maximum) |
| Brown's syndrome = 6 mm | |

### Operative Procedure

The superior oblique tendon is isolated using a temporal conjunctival incision with nasal tendon isolation, as described in the previous section (Figures 19.1 to 19.6). It is imperative to maintain the integrity of nasal intermuscular septum.

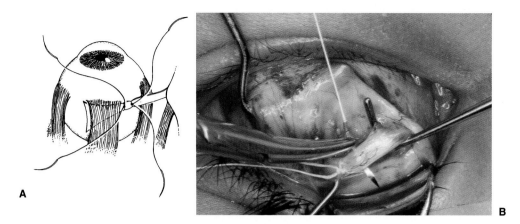

**FIGURE 19.9. (A)** Two 5-0 Mersilene double-arm sutures on spatula needles are secured to the superior oblique tendon. The first suture is placed 3 mm nasal to the superior rectus muscle, and the suture is secured by a full tendon width / half thickness pass through the superior oblique tendon. Two locking bites are placed at each edge of the tendon, and a square knot is made to tie the ends of the double arm suture together. The second 5-0 Mersilene suture is secured in a similar manner, 2 mm nasal to the first suture. **(B)** The needle is being passed through the superior oblique tendon to secure the first of two 5-0 Mersilene sutures to tendon.

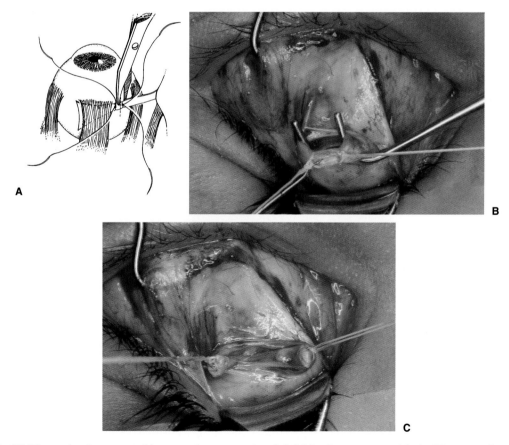

**FIGURE 19.10. (A)** The tendon is transected between the two preplaced 5-0 Mersilene sutures with the Westcott scissors. Exaggerated forced ductions of the superior oblique tendon should be performed to verify that the entire tendon has been severed (see Figure 10.23). **(B)** Two 5-0 Mersilene double arm sutures are secured to the tendon with the ends on stretch to expose the tendon between the sutures. **(C)** The cut ends of the superior oblique tendon have been secured with a 5-0 Mersilene suture. Notice that the cut ends of the tendon appear within the superior oblique fascial capsule. The nasal intermuscular septum, and floor of the superior oblique tendon capsule, remain intact.

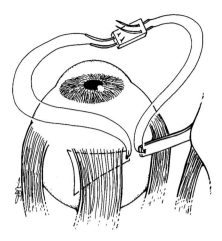

**FIGURE 19.11.** A medical-grade silicone 240 or 40 retinal band is presoaked in an antibiotic solution, and cut to the desired length. The double-arm sutures from the cut ends of the superior oblique tendon are then passed in a horizontal mattress fashion through the segment of silicone band.

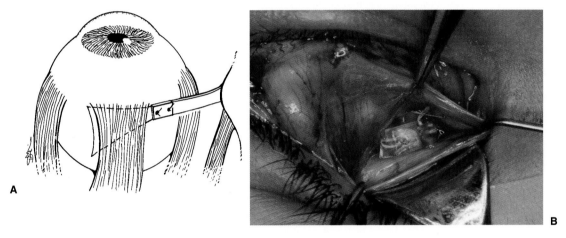

**FIGURE 19.12.** (A) The sutures are withdrawn from the silicone, and the silicone band is positioned between the cut ends of the tendon. The double-arm sutures are tied together, and excess sutures are removed. (B) The silicone band tied in place. The tendon capsule under the silicone is intact. The capsule and conjunctiva are separately closed over the silicone band with 6-0 plain gut suture. Careful closure of the capsule is important to prevent extrusion.

## Split Tendon Elongation

The split tendon elongation has the advantage of producing a graded elongation of the tendon without placing a foreign body such as a silicone retinal band. It is a little tricky to suture the tendon but can be mastered. Use the same technique as described above, for tendon exposure, in Figures 19.1 to 19.6.

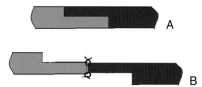

**FIGURE 19.13.** Diagram shows the split tendon elongation procedure. Note the tendon is split and the cut ends are tied together. Three millimeters of tendon split will result in 6 mm of separation. (**A**) Tendon is split for 3 to 4 mm. (**B**) Each end of split tendon is secured with a 5-0 Mersilene suture, then the ends are tied together to elongate the tendon.

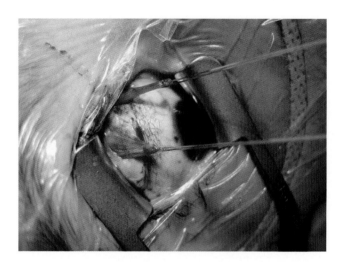

**FIGURE 19.14.** Photograph shows the superior oblique tendon after the split. The sutures are attached to the split tendon. The sutures are tied together to unite the tendon ends.

## Posterior Tenectomy

The selective removal of the posterior two-thirds of the tendon fibers will improve mild superior oblique overaction. Because the superior rectus muscle overlies the superior oblique tendon, simple posterior tenotomy is not very effective. The cut tendon fibers do not retract as they are held in place by overlying superior rectus muscle.

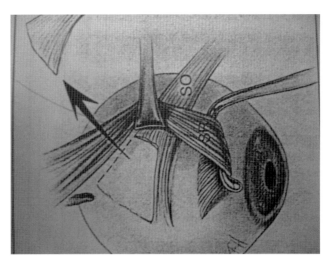

FIGURE 19.15. A posterior tenectomy is shown with removal of posterior two-thirds of the tendon fibers.

## Complications

Residual superior oblique overaction is probably the most common complication of superior oblique weakening procedures. This is often caused by missing the superior oblique tendon. The exaggerated forced duction maneuver, described by Guyton, should be performed after superior oblique tenotomy, to verify that the complete tendon has been severed (see Chapter 10). Missed fibers yield a positive exaggerated forced duction test. Standard forced ductions testing will not consistently identify missed superior oblique tendon fibers.

An infrequent complication is the misidentification of the superior rectus muscle as the superior oblique tendon. When the superior rectus is hooked and forcefully retracted, the superior rectus muscle blanches and looks remarkably similar to the superior oblique tendon.

When performing the Wright's silicone tendon expander, keep the floor of the superior oblique tendon capsule and nasal intermuscular septum intact. If the capsule floor is violated, the silicone implant will scar to sclera, producing an abnormal insertion. If the silicone scars anterior to the equator of the eye, it can cause postoperative limitation of depression.

Superior oblique palsy after superior oblique tenotomy is also a potential complication. Usually the paresis is mild if the intermuscular septum surrounding the tendon is left intact. This is not true, however, for patients with Brown's syndrome, as secondary superior oblique palsy after tenotomy occurs quite frequently. In patients with bilateral superior oblique overaction and good fusion, tenotomy should be avoided, as postoperative cyclovertical diplopia can occur. Patients at high risk for developing a consecutive superior oblique palsy and diplopia should have the Wright's silicone tendon expander procedure, which can provide better control over the amount of superior oblique weakening.

# 20 Faden Operation (Posterior Fixation Suture)

The faden operation, also termed *posterior fixation suture*, is used to weaken the rotational force of a rectus muscle when the eye rotates towards the faden muscle. Faden is the German word for suture, so it is inappropriate to call the procedure "faden suture" (i.e., suture-suture).

## How a Faden Works

The faden procedure is performed by suturing the rectus muscle to sclera, 12mm to 14mm posterior to the rectus muscle insertion. This pins the rectus muscle to the sclera so when the eye rotates towards the fadened muscle, the arc of contact cannot unravel. The faden suture thus creates a new insertion posterior to the original insertion. This posterior insertion shortens the moment arm when the eye rotates towards the fadened muscle. Shortening the moment arm reduces the rotational force as the eye rotates towards the fadened muscle (Figure 20.1).

## Indications for Faden Operation

In most cases, the faden operation is combined with a recession, as the effect of the faden operation by itself is relatively small. The faden operation works best on the medial rectus muscle because the medial rectus muscle has the shortest arc of contact (6mm). The short arc of contact of the medial rectus muscle is dramatically changed by a 12mm to 14mm faden. Alternately, the lateral rectus muscle is not affected very much by the faden because the arc of contact is 10mm, and pinning the muscle at 12mm to 14mm does not significantly change this naturally long arc of contact. Therefore, the faden operation is usually indicated to correct incomitance found with esotropia, by enhancing the effect of a medial rectus recession.

### Sixth Nerve Paresis

An example of where the faden may be most effective is with a partial sixth nerve palsy. The standard surgery has historically been a recession of the medial rectus muscle and resection of the lateral rectus muscle on the paretic eye. This helps correct the esodeviation in primary position, but does not address the large esotropia that occurs to the side of the paretic eye. A faden operation of the contralateral medial rectus muscle (yoke muscle to the paretic lateral rectus muscle) could improve this lateral incomitance. An alternative to the standard ipsilateral recession/resection is to add a small medial rectus recession with a faden to the contralateral

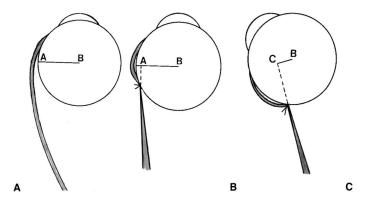

**FIGURE 20.1.** (**A**) This drawing shows the normal length of the moment arm when the eye is in primary position (line A-B). The moment arm equals the radius of the eye. (**B**) A faden pinning a rectus muscle 12 mm posterior to the muscle's insertion. The length of the moment arm remains unchanged with the eye in primary position (line A-B). (**C**) The eye rotated toward the fadened muscle. When the eye rotates towards the fadened muscle, the moment arm is significantly shortened (line C-B), because of the new posterior insertion site caused by the faden procedure. When the eye rotates away from the fadened muscle, the moment arm is the full radius of the eye. Thus the faden procedure only reduces rotational force when the eye moves towards the fadened muscle.

medial rectus muscle. A faden to the contralateral medial rectus muscle helps correct the esotropia that increases to the side of the paretic lateral rectus muscle by decreasing the rotational force of the yoke medial rectus, thus matching the paretic lateral rectus muscle. Matching yoke muscles only works if there is good lateral rectus function with only −1 to −2 limitation of abduction.

### High AC/A Ratio

The faden operation may be helpful when the patient has an esotropia with a high AC/A ratio. It is thought that the faden operation would reduce convergence at near, thus lowering the AC/A ratio. In these cases of high AC/A ratio esotropia, the option would be to perform bilateral medial rectus recessions along with the faden operation. Experience with this procedure indicates that it may reduce the AC/A ratio, however, most patients still require a bifocal add in order to obtain fusion at near. Presently, the use of a faden operation with a medial rectus recession in high AC/A ratio esotropia patients is controversial.

### Other Indications

Other indications for the faden operation have been reported including dissociated vertical deviation, nystagmus compensation syndrome, and nystagmus in primary position without a face turn. However, the efficacy of the faden operation in these situations has not been proven. In addition, some have advocated using the faden operation on the lateral rectus muscle in patients with Duane's retraction syndrome, and significant upshoot and downshoot. It is believed that the faden would pin the lateral rectus muscle so it would not slip above or below the eye, thus reducing the upshoot and downshoot.

## Surgical Techniques

### *Faden with Rectus Recession*

The faden operation requires extreme posterior exposure. It is important when performing a fornix incision, to extend the incision for approximately 4 mm to 5 mm over the area of the rectus muscle in order to obtain adequate posterior exposure (modified Swan).

The first aspect of the rectus muscle recession and faden procedure is to secure the rectus muscle and disinsert it from the sclera, as described for rectus recession in Chapters 10 and 11. Once the muscle is removed, the posterior fixation suture is placed through the sclera 12 mm to 14 mm posterior to the rectus muscle insertion in the center of the arc of contact. A nonabsorbable suture (e.g., 5-0 Dacron on the t-5 Alcon needle or a 5-0 Mersilene on a spatula needle) is preferred. It is important to use a spatula needle in order to help avoid scleral perforation.

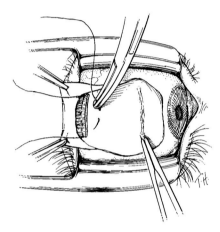

**FIGURE 20.2.** The drawing shows the recessed rectus muscle and a suture being placed 12 mm posterior to the scleral insertion through sclera in the middle of the muscle's arc of contact. Use a 5-0 Mersilene double arm suture with a spatula needle. A large posterior dissection, removing intermuscular septum and check ligaments, is important to obtain proper posterior exposure. Note that the suture is passed parallel with the scleral insertion line for a distance of 3 mm to 4 mm. The suture is then pulled through, and left in sclera with half the suture above and half the suture below the scleral pass. The rectus muscle is then attached to sclera at the appropriate recession point using standard scleral passes.

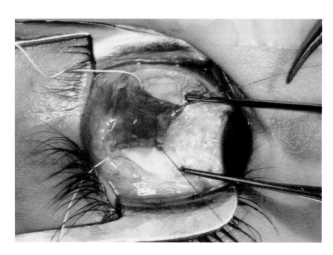

**FIGURE 20.3.** The rectus muscle is to be reattached to sclera with a recession of approximately 4 mm. Note the white Mersilene suture underlying the rectus muscle. This is a double arm suture with needles at each end of the Mersilene suture. Each half of the suture will be passed underneath the lateral one-third of the rectus muscle and tied over the rectus muscle to complete the mattress suture.

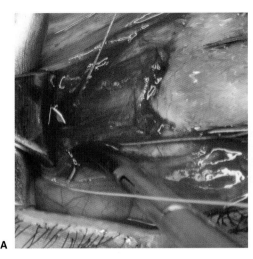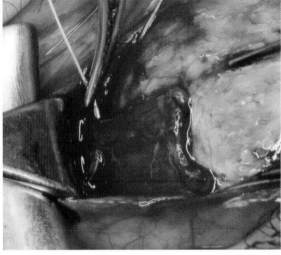

**FIGURE 20.4. (A)** A needle on the lower third of the rectus muscle is being passed in the direction from deep to superficial, to avoid scleral perforation. The muscle is secured 12 mm posterior to the muscle insertion. **(B)** The needle is being passed through the superior third of the muscle, again passing from deep to superficial, to avoid scleral perforation. The muscle is secured 12 mm posterior to the muscle insertion.

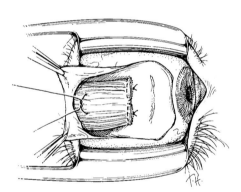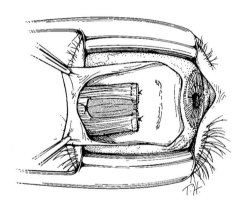

**FIGURE 20.5.** Tying the two ends of the 5-0 Mersilene suture together completes the central mattress suture. A surgeon's knot is tied firmly to secure the muscle to sclera. Do not overtighten, as it will cause necrosis of the anterior muscle. Make sure that all slack is taken out of the Mersilene mattress suture, as blind loops of suture can occur underneath the muscle.

**FIGURE 20.6.** The 5-0 Mersilene suture is tied in place with a rectus recession. Note that the darkened shaded area represents muscle fibers that are captured by the posterior fixation suture. These fibers are isolated and are not capable of exerting torque on the eye.

*Faden Without Recession*

It is infrequent that a faden operation is performed without a rectus recession. If there is very little deviation in primary position, however, this procedure may be indicated to correct lateral incomitance.

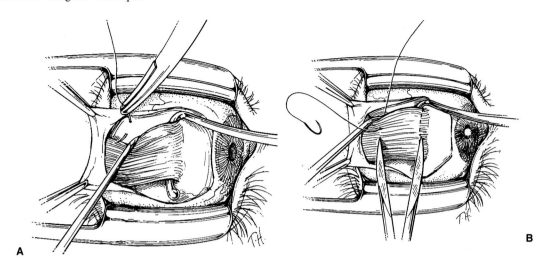

**FIGURE 20.7.** **(A)** The rectus muscle is isolated and secured with a muscle hook in the routine fashion using either the limbal approach or a fornix approach with extension of the incision over part of the rectus muscle. Be sure to perform an extensive posterior dissection of intermuscular septum and check ligaments to expose the muscle for approximately 14 mm posterior to the muscle insertion. Secure a single arm 5-0 Mersilene suture on a spatula needle through the sclera, 12 mm posterior to the muscle insertion at the border of the rectus muscle for a scleral pass of approximately 3 mm. **(B)** The same needle is being passed through the inferior 1/4 of the rectus muscle in a direction of deep to superficial. A separate suture is placed at both borders of the rectus muscle in a similar manner.

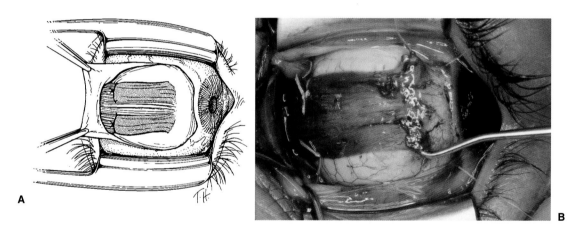

**FIGURE 20.8.** **(A)** Both sutures are tied in place incorporating the lateral one-fourth of each border of the rectus muscle 12 mm posterior to the muscle insertion. **(B)** The two Mersilene sutures are tied in place at the borders of the muscle. Note the Desmarres retractor being used to gain posterior exposure.

## Complications

Perhaps the most common complication of the faden procedure is lack of effect. A faden, by itself, has been shown to change muscle function minimally. In addition, one of the problems associated with performing the faden operation is to gain posterior access. In order to be effective, the suture must be placed 12 mm to 14 mm posterior to the muscle insertion. Making a generous conjunctival incision will help to obtain good exposure.

Another complication is muscle necrosis, occurring if the sutures are tied too tightly. In addition, patients can have scarring in the area of the faden if orbital fat is inadvertently exposed during the posterior dissection. Scleral perforation and retinal tear are always a risk in any strabismus surgery, but are especially important to consider in regards to the faden operation.

# 21  Reoperation Techniques

For most reoperations, standard recession and resection techniques can be used. The major difference from surgery on a virgin muscle is the need to mobilize the conjunctiva in front of and over the muscle. Reoperation for a lost muscle and strabismus after retinal detachment surgery, however, are situations that tend to be technically more difficult and require special techniques. This chapter will cover surgical approaches to muscle dehiscence, lost muscle, and strabismus occurring after retinal detachment surgery.

## Muscle Dehiscence: Lost Muscle

A muscle dehiscence is a separation of the muscle from its scleral attachment. There are three basic types of muscle dehiscence that have been identified, including slipped muscle, lost muscle, and stretched scar. The medial rectus muscle is the most commonly slipped or lost rectus muscle, and is also the most difficult to find because it has no oblique muscle connections, and it is free to retract posterior to the globe. There are oblique muscle attachments to the other rectus muscles that keep rectus muscles from retracting posterior to the globe: the superior rectus muscle to the superior oblique muscle, the lateral rectus muscle to the inferior oblique muscle, and the inferior rectus muscle to the inferior oblique muscle. In cases of slipped, or even most lost rectus muscles, there is usually a pseudotendon or fibrous scar from the previous scleral insertion site back to the slipped/lost muscle.

### Slipped Muscle

First described by Parks and Bloom in 1979, the slipped muscle occurs after inadequate suturing of muscle, resulting in muscle capsule attached to sclera, while the muscle itself retracts posteriorly.[1] Ductions are limited but relatively preserved, as compared to a lost muscle (Figure 21.1A). Plager and Parks described the crucial finding of the muscle recoiled posteriorly within the capsule, found at the Tenon's capsule penetration site.[2] They also described specific intraoperative findings of a translucent "empty, friable avascular capsule attached to the globe" (Figure 21.1B). A slipped muscle occurs immediately with the limited ductions usually identified within a day or two after strabismus surgery, but the slippage can continue over time. Treatment is retrieval, excision of capsule attachment, and advancement of the muscle to the intended surgical site with a nonabsorbable suture. Often the antagonist is contracted and tight, adding a restrictive component. If the antagonist is tight it should be recessed.

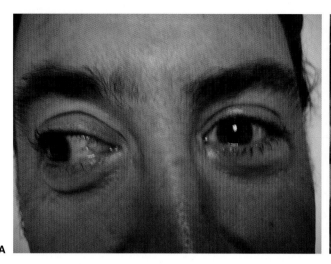
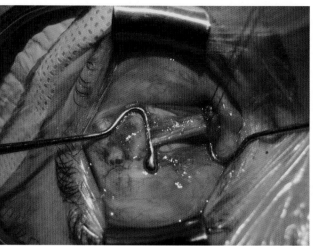

A

B

**FIGURE 21.1.** **(A)** Patient with a slipped left medial rectus muscle after medial rectus recession. Note that the patient is looking to the right demonstrating a large exotropia with the left eye showing limited adduction and lid fissure widening. **(B)** Surgical exploration shows a translucent avascular capsule connecting the globe to the medial rectus muscle. Note that the capsular attachment is so thin you can see the large Jameson hook through the overlying capsule.

*Lost Muscle*

The lost muscle has long been a dreaded complication of periocular surgery including pterygium surgery, retinal detachment surgery, and strabismus surgery. A lost rectus muscle can occur when a muscle is surgically removed from the globe, or it can be associated with the pulled in two syndrome (PITS) when the muscle is torn in two by pulling too hard on the muscle. PITS is more common in elderly patients, and can occur with relatively minimal muscle traction. The hallmark of a lost muscle is severely limited ductions and palpebral fissure widening on attempted gaze in the direction of the lost muscle. The treatment is exploration and retrieval of the lost muscle. If the muscle cannot be found immediately during the primary surgery, it is often best to wait two weeks to perform the secondary exploration surgery. By waiting to reoperate the swelling subsides and a fibrous scar usually forms, which extends from the scleral insertion to the site of the lost muscle. This scar can be traced posteriorly, to help find a lost muscle (see Figures 21.2 to 21.9). Once the lost muscle is found, secure and reattach the muscle with nonabsorbable suture. The antagonist to the lost muscle is usually contracted and tight. If diagnosed tight by forced ductions, recess the tight antagonist. If the lost muscle cannot be found, a rectus muscle transposition is indicated, with a large recession of the antagonist muscle.

*Stretched Scar*

Stretched scar is a lengthening of the muscle to sclera fibrous attachment that occurs several weeks to months after strabismus surgery. This results in posterior retraction of the muscle and reduced muscle function. In 1999, Ludwig first described this phenomenon as a common cause of unfavorable outcomes after strabismus surgery.[3] Using an animal model, Ludwig showed that muscles sutured with an absorbable suture had a significantly higher rate of stretched scar than those sutured with a nonabsorbable suture. Ludwig hypothesized that the mechanism of stretched scar is weakening of the absorbable suture before the muscle to sclera healing is complete. Like slipped muscle, patients with stretched scar have an amorphous fibrous band connecting the muscle to the globe, however, the tissue is thicker with a stretched scar (see Figures 21.10 and 21.11). Also similar to a slipped muscle, ductions are limited but less limited than a lost muscle. In contrast to a slipped muscle that occurs immediately, stretched scar occurs late, at least 4 to 6 weeks after surgery. Treatment is excision of scar and advancement using a non-absorbable suture to secure the muscle to the intended insertion site (see Figures 21.12 to 21.14). Add a recession of the antagonist muscle if it is tight on forced duction testing.

## Surgery for a Lost Medial Rectus Muscle

Figures 21.2 to 21.9 show the surgical approach to a lost left medial rectus muscle. The author has developed a conjunctival incision that is a combination of the fornix and Swan incisions. This allows immediate access to the posterior aspect of the quadrant between the muscles to allow hooking of the muscle or its scar, and great exposure of the area over the muscle. This incision also avoids having to mobilize the bulbar conjunctiva in front of the muscle that is usually scarred to sclera. Postoperative appearance of the conjunctiva is quite good with this technique.

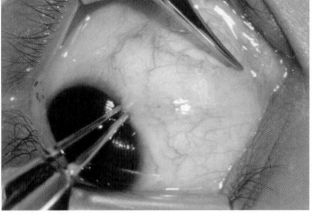

**FIGURE 21.2.** A blunt curved Westcott scissors is used to make an incision in the inferior nasal fornix through conjunctiva. After the conjunctival incision, use the Westcott scissors and spread into the inferior nasal quadrant, keeping the scissors tips down on sclera to remove adhesions to sclera. The conjunctiva may be adherent to sclera, requiring blunt and sharp dissection to mobilize the conjunctiva.

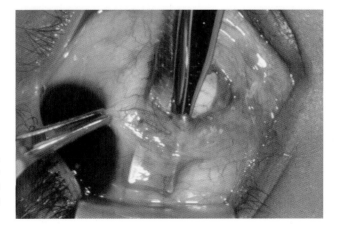

**FIGURE 21.3.** After the quadrant is open and free of adhesions, undermine the conjunctiva in front of the area of medial rectus insertion site by spreading the blunt Westcott scissors as shown in the figure. Firm conjunctival–scleral adhesions are removed with sharp dissection staying close to sclera.

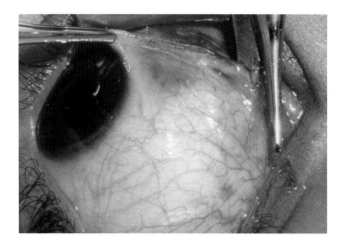

**FIGURE 21.4.** Once the conjunctiva anterior to the original muscle insertion is mobilized, perform a Swan incision, by extending the conjunctival incision superiorly over the area of the muscle insertion as shown. Be sure to keep the incision in front of the plica and semilunar folds.

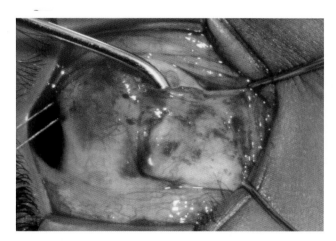

**FIGURE 21.5.** Secure the muscle (or muscle scar) by passing a small hook in the inferior nasal quadrant, orienting the hook perpendicular on bare sclera, and then passing the hook underneath the tissue where the medial rectus muscle insertion should be based on the previous surgery. This pass of the small Stevens hook should be made at least 5 mm posterior to the presumed insertion site. Once tissue is hooked with the small Stevens hook, pass a von Graefe hook behind the small hook, and then remove the small hook. The von Graefe hook has a smooth end (no foot or bulb), so it is easier to pass under a scarred muscle than the Green or Jameson hooks. The photograph shows the von Graefe hook behind a fibrovascular tissue that could possibly be the muscle or a scar to the slipped muscle. A scar that connects and attaches sclera to a slipped muscle is termed the "pseudotendon." Note that in the photograph, there is a Vicryl traction suture placed at the limbus, pulling the eye out laterally, aiding with exposure. Be sure not to pull too hard on the Von Graefe hook as the pseudotendon can rupture.

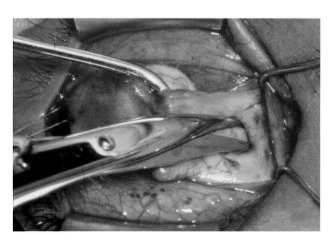

**FIGURE 21.6.** Figure shows spreading action with the Westcott scissors used to dissect posteriorly over the presumed pseudotendon to follow it through the muscle sleeve in search of the slipped muscle. Blunt and sharp dissection with the Westcott scissors is used to follow the scar posteriorly as it penetrates a scarred muscle sleeve. Note that the curved Westcott scissors are tip down to avoid penetration into surrounding extraconal orbital fat. Mild countertraction by the von Graefe hook keeps the pseudotendon on stretch. A 6-0 Vicryl traction suture at the limbus is still in place, helping to keep the eye abducted and to gain posterior exposure without having to pull too hard with the von Graefe hook.

**FIGURE 21.7.** Further dissection along the pseudotendon involves removing scarred intermuscular septum. In the photograph, the inferior intermuscular septum is thickened and scarred to the sides of the pseudotendon, and is removed with a curved blunt Westcott scissors pointed tip down. Dissect close to the pseudotendon to avoid penetration of Tenon's capsule and exposure of orbital fat. Manipulation of orbital fat can lead to fat adherence syndrome and postoperative restriction. If fat is inadvertently exposed, close the tear in Tenon's capsule with 7-0 Vicryl to cover and isolate the fat. Note that two small Stevens hooks are used to retract the muscle sleeve and gain posterior exposure. Each side of the pseudotendon is cleared of scarred intermuscular septum.

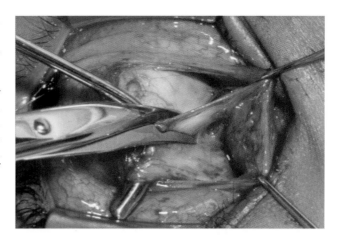

**FIGURE 21.8.** The dissection has been performed along the pseudotendon approximately 12 mm posterior to the insertion site, or around 20 mm posterior to the limbus. Note the pinkish-white scar tissue extends posteriorly to join a dark brown tissue in the area of the Desmarres retractor. This dark brown tissue at the posterior aspect of the pseudotendon is the true medial rectus muscle *(see arrow)*. At this point it is clear that the scar tissue followed posteriorly was not muscle, but is a pseudotendon (fibrovascular scar connected to the slipped muscle). The Desmarres retractor works well to retract the muscle sleeve and gain posterior exposure.

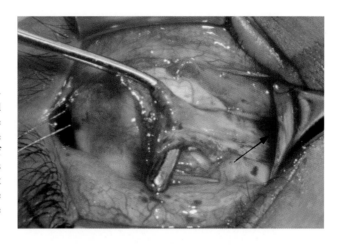

**FIGURE 21.9.** Photograph taken after further securing the true medial rectus muscle with a double arm suture. The muscle is secured with a central security knot and locking bites at each edge. We now use a nonabsorbable 5-0 Mersilene suture to prevent a slipped muscle or stretched scar. The central security knot is applied as soon as the true muscle is identified because the pseudotendon can inadvertently tear at any time. After the security knot is placed, the muscle is secured in the routine fashion with locking bites at each edge of the muscle.

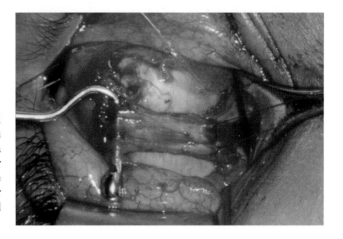

Once the muscle is secured. the pseudotendon is resected and the muscle is advanced, usually to a position close to the original insertion. Lost/slipped rectus muscles are contracted and tight so be sure to make secure scleral passes to avoid sutures pulling out of sclera. In these cases of lost/slipped rectus muscles it is difficult to predict postoperative alignment. Try the spring-back forced duction balance testing at the time of surgery, by rotating the eye back and forth and then releasing to find the position of rest of the eye. Another option is to use the adjustable suture technique, however, because of postoperative drift and the difficulty of adjustment on a reoperation patient, the author rarely uses adjustable sutures. If an adjustable suture is used, place the recessed antagonist on an adjustable suture. Do not place the advanced lost/slipped muscle on an adjustable suture as it is very tight and may slip postoperatively.

## Surgery for Stretched Scar

The following is a description of the approach to a reoperation for a stretched scar left medial rectus muscle.

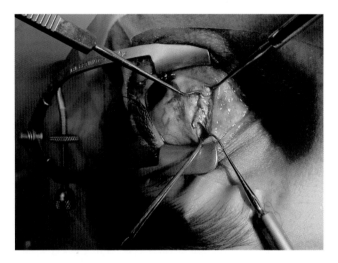

**FIGURE 21.10.** The left medial rectus muscle has been hooked through a combination fornix-Swan incision. At first look the muscle appears to be appropriately inserting at the intended recession point.

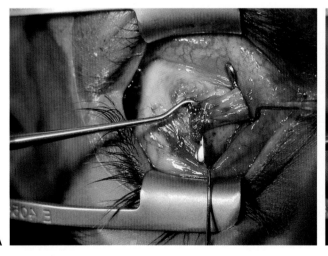
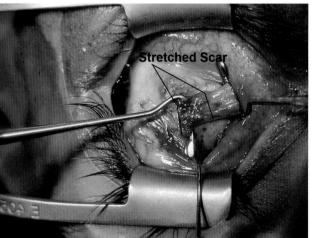

A                                                                                                              B

**FIGURE 21.11.** **(A)** Dissection of the medial rectus discloses the muscle. Note the anterior 4 mm to 5 mm of the muscle has a different appearance than the posterior muscle fibers. **(B)** The lines indicate the area of stretched scar (5 mm to 6 mm). The true muscle fibers are located 5 mm to 6 mm posterior to the scleral insertion.

**FIGURE 21.12.** The true muscle fibers are secured with a nonabsorbable suture, with a central security knot and full thickness locking bites at each edge of the muscle. The area of stretched scar anterior to the sutures is excised. There is no significant bleeding with scar excision.

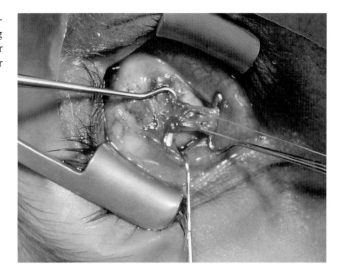

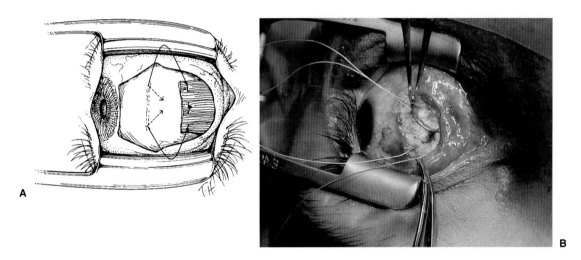

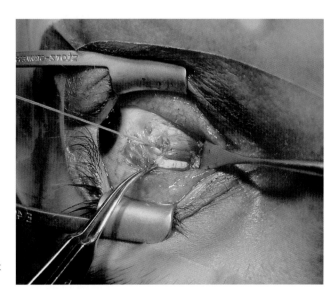

**FIGURE 21.13.** (A) Drawing shows the scleral needle passes directed posterior to the insertion. This technique of the posterior needle passes places the suture knot under the advanced muscle. By keeping the knot posterior and under the muscle it reduces the chances of late knot erosion through the conjunctiva. (B) Companion photograph showing the needles in sclera directed posteriorly away from the cornea.

**FIGURE 21.14.** The muscle is advanced and tied in place. The knot is under the muscle.

## Pearls for Reoperation: Rectus Dehiscence–Lost Muscle

1. The combination Fornix Swan incision is useful for isolating previously operated rectus muscles. First perform a fornix incision to access bare sclera. Then use the blunt Westcott scissors to spread in the quadrant to remove scar. Next, hook the rectus muscle with a small Stevens hook followed by a large Jameson hook. Once the muscle is secured extend the conjunctival incision over the muscle insertion as per a Swan incision.

2. Do not dissect posteriorly directly on sclera to look for a slipped/lost medial rectus muscle. A lost or slipped medial rectus muscle will retract within the muscle sleeve, and will be surrounded by orbital fat. A lost/slipped medial rectus muscle is usually found within the muscle sleeve as shown above. Posterior dissection along sclera can be dangerous as the optic nerve can be inadvertently damaged or removed as it is only approximately 22 mm posterior to the nasal limbus.

3. A lost lateral rectus muscle can almost always be found by exploring the inferior oblique muscle insertion. The lateral rectus muscle has strong attachments to the inferior oblique insertion, and a lost lateral rectus muscle will retract to the inferior oblique insertion.

4. Use nonabsorbable sutures to reduce the chances of a secondary stretched scar.

## Strabismus after Retinal Detachment Surgery

### Causes of Strabismus

The incidence of strabismus after retinal surgery is between 3% and 20%, depending on the study referenced. Transient diplopia associated with a small angle strabismus immediately after retinal detachment surgery is common and usually resolves spontaneously within a few weeks. Patients with bothersome diplopia that persists longer than 4 to 6 months should be considered for strabismus surgery.

Strabismus is usually caused by periocular fibrosis and fat adherence. Shortened conjunctiva and subconjunctival fibrosis also contribute to the restriction and strabismus. An encircling retinal band does not significantly alter rectus muscle function, and this is why, in the majority of cases, the scleral buckle procedures do not cause strabismus. Large diameter implants such as silicone sponges placed directly underneath a muscle can, however, deflect the muscle's course, and tighten a muscle causing restriction. Other causes of strabismus include entrapment of an oblique muscle by encircling elements.

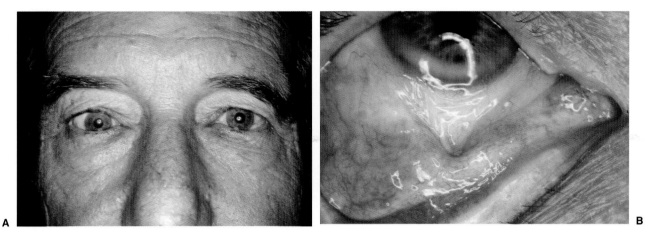

FIGURE 21.15. (A) A patient with a right hypotropia and esotropia after a scleral buckle procedure for the right eye. Eversion of the lower lid shows thickened conjunctiva, indicating fat adherence, which is anterior to the inferior rectus insertion. (B) In addition, the conjunctiva is shortened and scarred, thus pulling the eye down. This patient is an example of restrictive strabismus secondary to fat adherence, periocular fibrosis, and conjunctival scarring.

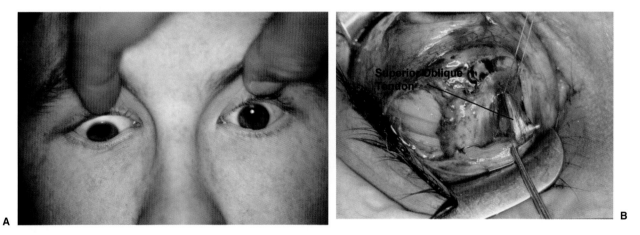

FIGURE 21.16. (A) A patient with severe limitation of depression, left eye, immediately after a 360° encircling element is shown. (B) Exploration of the superior rectus muscle and superior oblique tendon. This revealed that the superior oblique tendon had been entrapped by the scleral buckle and displaced anteriorly to the nasal border of the superior rectus muscle insertion. In the photograph the superior oblique tendon is hooked with a small Stevens hook, and is found inserted at the nasal aspect of the superior rectus insertion. A 6-0 Vicryl suture (purple suture) has been secured to the superior oblique tendon at its new insertion next to the superior rectus insertion. Note the large encircling element under the superior rectus muscle. This anterior insertion of the superior oblique causes limited depression. The superior oblique tendon in this case was replaced posterior to the retinal band, resulting in dramatic improvement of the restriction in down gaze.

## Surgical Approach for Strabismus after Retinal Detachment Surgery

The goal of surgery is to first identify the cause or causes of the restriction. Forced ductions at the time of surgery is helpful in identifying the area of restriction. It should be performed with and without retropulsion of the eye. Retropulsion of the eye slackens the rectus muscle and, if forced ductions improve with retropulsion, then the restriction is secondary to a tight rectus muscle. Persistent restriction after retropulsion of the eye indicates that periocular scarring or oblique muscle restriction is contributing to the restriction. In most cases of strabismus after retinal surgery, there are significant periocular adhesions. As a result, the ductions are limited both with and without retropulsion of the eye. Once an area of restriction is identified, it is surgically explored. Scar in the area causing the restriction is removed. The appropriate rectus muscle in the area of restriction is identified, secured with a suture, and then detached from sclera. Forced ductions are repeated to verify that the restriction is released. The detached rectus muscle is reattached to the globe recessing the muscle, usually using an adjustable suture technique appropriate to correct the strabismus. Often, a vertical and horizontal strabismus will coexist. In these cases a vertical and horizontal rectus muscle will have to be recessed.

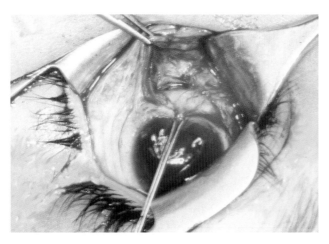

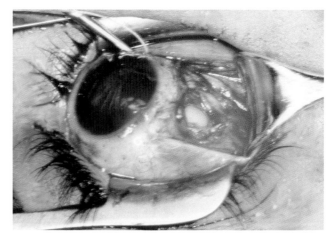

FIGURE 21.17. Patient with esotropia and severe restriction to abduction after retinal detachment surgery. Surgical exploration of the left medial rectus muscle through an inferior nasal fornix incision. Photograph shows exposure of inferior nasal quadrant and the anterior portion of the encircling band. A traction suture of 5-0 Mersilene has been placed at the limbus to pull the eye up and out, thus exposing the inferior nasal quadrant. Once the scleral buckle is identified, it can be followed superiorly to help find the medial rectus muscle. Because of scarring, the medial rectus muscle may be hard to identify. To help find a rectus muscle, pass a small Stevens hook or a von Graefe hook along the scleral buckle under the area where the muscle is supposed to be. Because the buckle passes behind the rectus muscles, the buckle will help in identifying the rectus muscle insertion. Note that the Desmarres retractor is useful for gaining posterior exposure.

FIGURE 21.18. A von Graefe hook is behind the left medial rectus muscle and scar. This hook was passed along the scleral buckle as the scleral buckle courses underneath the rectus muscle. A decrease in the heart rate (vasovagal reflex) indicates that the muscle was hooked. Dissection on either side of the muscle hook reveals muscle encapsulated in scar. This muscle was recessed en bloc with the posterior scar left on the muscle. Dissecting the posterior scar off the muscle can lead to further scarring and fat adherence. Removal of adhesions and recession of the medial rectus muscle released the restriction.

## Pearls for Strabismus after Retinal Detachment Surgery

1. When dissecting to remove periocular adhesions, dissect close to sclera to avoid violating orbital fat. Be careful of posterior dissections, especially along the nasal aspect of the globe, as cases of inadvertent removal of the optic nerve have occurred. Dissection of scar must be performed under direct visualization.

2. The muscle can be recessed by a hang-back technique, hanging the muscle back over the silicone-encircling element. Use a nonabsorbable suture to reduce the chances of a postoperative stretched scar, and to help retrieval of the muscle if another surgery is necessary. In most cases, it is not necessary to remove the scleral buckle. If the scleral buckle appears to be unstable, or is exposed at the time of strabismus surgery, it can be removed, usually without significantly increasing the risk of redetachment as long as the buckle has been in place for several months. Before surgery, it is best to consult with the patient's retinal surgeon in regards to safety of removing the buckle.

3. At the end of the case the conjunctiva should be recessed in the area of the restriction. The anterior sclera should be carefully cleared of scar and fibrosis, leaving the sclera smooth so postoperative reepithelialization can occur without resulting in a chronic red eye. Careful suturing of the conjunctiva is important to avoid postoperative sub-conjunctival cysts. The author prefers 6-0 plain gut suture for conjunctival closure.

## References

1. Parks MM, Bloom JN. The "slipped muscle." Ophthalmology 1979;86:1389–1396.
2. Plager DA, Parks MM. Recognition and repair of the "lost" rectus muscle. A report of 25 cases. Ophthalmology 1990;97:131–136; discussion 136–137.
3. Ludwig IH. Scar remodeling after strabismus surgery. Trans Am Ophthalmol Soc 1999;97:583–651.

# Appendixes

# Appendix I
## Surgical Numbers

The following tables can be used as a guideline in planning strabismus surgery. These numbers have been derived from Parks, with modifications from the surgical experience of the author. The numbers are only a guide and should be modified as necessary.

### Binocular Surgery

*Esotropia*

| MR OU Recession | LR OU Resection* |
|---|---|
| $15^\Delta$—3.0 mm | $15^\Delta$—3.5 mm |
| $20^\Delta$—3.5 mm | $20^\Delta$—4.5 mm |
| $25^\Delta$—4.0 mm | $25^\Delta$—5.5 mm |
| $30^\Delta$—4.5 mm | $30^\Delta$—6.0 mm |
| $35^\Delta$—5.0 mm | $35^\Delta$—6.5 mm |
| $40^\Delta$—5.5 mm | $40^\Delta$—7.0 mm |
| $50^\Delta$—6.0 mm | $50^\Delta$—8.0 mm |
| $60^\Delta$—6.5 mm | |
| $70^\Delta$—7.0 mm | |

* When a lateral rectus resection is done for residual esotropia after a large medial rectus recession (6.0 mm or larger), these numbers should be lowered.

*Exotropia*

| LR OU Recession | MR OU Resection |
|---|---|
| $15^\Delta$—4.0 mm | $15^\Delta$—3.0 mm |
| $20^\Delta$—5.0 mm | $20^\Delta$—4.0 mm |
| $25^\Delta$—6.0 mm | $25^\Delta$—5.0 mm |
| $30^\Delta$—7.0 mm | $30^\Delta$—5.5 mm |
| $35^\Delta$—7.5 mm | $35^\Delta$—6.0 mm |
| $40^\Delta$—8.0 mm | $40^\Delta$—6.5 mm |
| $50^\Delta$—9.0 mm | |

## Monocular Surgery

*Esotropia*

| MR Recession | LR Resection |
|---|---|
| $15^\Delta$—3.0 mm | 3.5 mm |
| $20^\Delta$—3.5 mm | 4.0 mm |
| $25^\Delta$—4.0 mm | 5.0 mm |
| $30^\Delta$—4.5 mm | 5.5 mm |
| $35^\Delta$—5.0 mm | 6.0 mm |
| $40^\Delta$—5.5 mm | 6.5 mm |
| $50^\Delta$—6.0 mm | 7.0 mm |
| $60^\Delta$—6.5 mm | 7.5 mm |
| $70^\Delta$—7.0 mm | 8.0 mm |

*Exotropia*

| LR Recession | MR Resection |
|---|---|
| $15^\Delta$—4.0 mm | 3.0 mm |
| $20^\Delta$—5.0 mm | 4.0 mm |
| $25^\Delta$—6.0 mm | 4.5 mm |
| $30^\Delta$—6.5 mm | 5.0 mm |
| $35^\Delta$—7.0 mm | 5.5 mm |
| $40^\Delta$—7.5 mm | 6.0 mm |
| $50^\Delta$—8.5 mm | 6.5 mm |

## Three Muscle Surgery

For large amounts of correction, surgery on three muscles may be planned for the primary operation. The amount of surgery can be judged from the above tables. This works especially well in adults, where one muscle can be placed on an adjustable suture. The adjustable suture should be done on the eye for which two muscles are being operated.

## Vertical Numbers

A rule of thumb for vertical surgery is 3 prism diopters of vertical correction for every millimeter of recession. Inferior rectus recessions are notorious for late overcorrections therefore, under most circumstances, do not recess the inferior rectus muscle more than 5 mm to 6 mm. Superior rectus recessions for dissociated vertical deviation (DVD), on the other hand, must be large, with the minimum recession of approximately 5 mm and a maximum of 9 mm (fixed suture technique).

## Kestenbaum Procedure for Nystagmus

### Face turn to the RIGHT

To correct the right face turn (eyes shifted to a left null point), move the eyes to primary position by moving both eyes to the right.

| | | LEFT EYE | | RIGHT EYE | |
| --- | --- | --- | --- | --- | --- |
| | Degree of Face Turn | Recess LR | Resect MR | Recess MR | Resect LR |
| **Classic** | <20° | 7 mm | 6 mm | 5 mm | 8 mm |
| **Parks** | 30° | 9 mm | 8 mm | 6.5 mm | 10 mm |
| *Classic +40%* | 45° | 10 mm | 8.5 mm | 7 mm | 11 mm |
| *Classic +60%* | 50° | 11 mm | 9.5 mm | 8 mm | 12.5 mm |

# Appendix II
## Anesthesia

General anesthesia is used most frequently in strabismus surgery. All surgery on children requires general anesthesia. Patient anxiety, re-operations, and superior oblique surgery are also indications for general anesthesia. An experienced anesthesiologist, familiar with pediatric anesthesia and potential life-threatening complications like malignant hyperthermia, is an essential member of the surgical team. Paralyzing anesthetic agents are not required.

Local anesthesia can be used in cooperative adults for unilateral surgery. A routine retrobulbar injection of 4 ml of lidocaine is given with a semi-blunt retrobulbar needle. If the patient experiences intraoperative pain, it can be treated with an additional, local injection of lidocaine near the muscle, being careful not to inject directly into the muscle itself. Retrobulbar anesthesia is most useful for recession—plication (or resection) procedures, usually for sensory strabismus.

Topical anesthesia is a good option for adult patients requiring a recession procedure unilateral or bilateral, although some even use topical anesthesia for resections and simple reoperations. With gentle manipulation of the tissues and avoiding pulling on the muscle, topical anesthesia strabismus surgery can be done with no or minimal pain, without bearing the risks of general anesthesia. (Refer to Chapter 12 for Topical Anesthesia Strabismus Surgery.)

# Appendix III
## Instruments for Muscle Surgery

| A | Stevens hook (3) <br> Green hook (2) <br> Jameson hook (2) <br> Von Graefe hook, large (1) |
|---|---|
| B | Conway retractor (1) <br> Desmarres retractor, medium (1) <br> Desmarres retractor, large (1) |
| C | Blunt Westcott scissors (1) |
| D | Bishop Harman forceps (2) <br> 2 × 3 Lester forceps (1) <br> Castroviejo forceps 0.3 (2) <br> Castroviejo forceps 0.5 (1) <br> Castroviejo locking forceps (2) |
| E | Castroviejo caliper (1) |
| F | Serrefine clamp (4) <br> Hartman clamp (2) |
| G | Superior oblique tendon tucker |
| | Wright titanium instruments <br> (see figures H1 to H4) |
| H1 <br> H2 <br> H3 <br> H4 | Wright grooved hook (1) (Titan Surgical OE018.01) <br> Wright double hook (1) (Titan Surgical OE018.02) <br> Wright bladed lid speculum (1) (Titan Surgical OR005) <br> Wright curved needle holder, carbide tip, locking/ <br> unlocking handle (1) (Titan Surgical 0H050U) |

## Sutures

A 5-0 Vicryl suture with S-24 double-arm spatula needles, or a 6-0 Vicryl suture with S-29 spatula needles, are the usual sutures of choice for strabismus surgery. The author, at the time of this book, prefers the 5-0 Vicryl suture. A 5-0 Mersilene suture (nonabsorbable suture) is indicated for muscles that may develop a postoperative stretched scar such as a thyroid inferior rectus muscle, advancement of a slipped muscle, the Harada-Ito procedure, and Wright's silicone tendon expander procedure.

## Magnification Light Source

A head lamp is advised, especially for oblique surgery. Magnification of 2 times is also helpful, but high magnification should be avoided as it significantly limits depth of focus and field size.

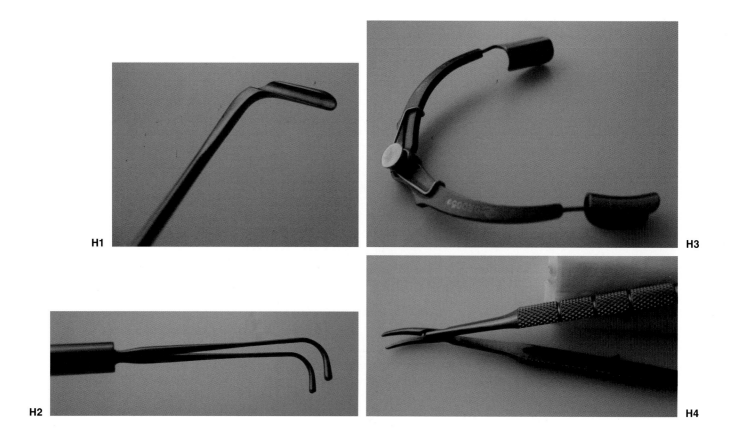

H1

H3

H2

H4

# Appendix IV
## Postoperative Care

**A**. Immediate Recovery

1. NPO for 1 to 2 hours after surgery, depending on the age of the patient. Restricting all oral intake helps reduce nausea and vomiting postoperatively. It is the author's experience that oral fluids given immediately after strabismus surgery result in a high incidence of nausea and vomiting.

2. Do not use eye patches unless an adjustable suture was used or it was a multiple reoperation.

**B**. Outpatient Follow-up

1. Prescribe antibiotic-steroid ointment, b.i.d. x four days.
2. No swimming for two weeks.
3. Schedule a follow-up post-op visit in the first week, then a second post-op visit usually in six weeks. This is extremely variable and depends on the patient's condition and age. Young patients operated for intermittent exotropia, who are initially overcorrected, need to be followed more frequently. Patients should be warned of the possibility of periocular infection and to return immediately if redness or swelling persists.

# Index

Printed in Singapore